Research Strategies
in Human Communication
Disorders

Research Strategies in Human Communication Disorders

Second Edition

Donald G. Doehring

pro·ed

8700 Shoal Creek Boulevard
Austin, Texas 78757-6897

pro·ed

©1996, 1988 by PRO-ED, Inc.
8700 Shoal Creek Boulevard
Austin, Texas 78757-6897

Library of Congress Cataloging-in-Publication Data

Doehring, Donald G.
    Research strategies in human communication disorders / Donald G.
    Doehring. — 2nd ed.
        p.   cm.
    Includes bibliographical references and index.
    ISBN 0-89079-644-0 (pbk.)
    1. Communicative disorders—Research—Methodology.   I. Title.
RC429.D64   1996
616.85'5'0072—dc20   95-44288
                                                                                      CIP

This book is designed in Fenice and Goudy.

Production Manager: Alan Grimes
Production Coordinator: Karen Swain
Managing Editor: Tracy Sergo
Art Director: Thomas Barkley
Reprints Buyer: Alicia Woods
Editor: Sue Motzer
Editorial Assistant: Claudette Landry
Editorial Assistant: Martin Wilson

Printed in the United States of America

1   2   3   4   5   6   7   8   9   10   00   99   98   97   96

Contents

Preface

This revised edition of *Research Strategies in Human Communication Disorders* once again describes the methods used in standard group research designs, and has a greatly expanded discussion of other research designs.

Part I describes the group research methods most commonly used in research in human communication disorders. It is intended for readers who have little or no previous experience regarding research methods, and also for those who wish to review their previous knowledge in the context of human communication disorders research. Equal attention is paid to research design and data analysis. Review questions and exercises are included for help in understanding special terms, concepts, and methods.

Part II describes other research methods, including observational, case study, and descriptive methods; statistical power analysis, meta-analysis, and multiple methods; single subject designs; qualitative methods; and path analysis, maximum likelihood estimation, loglinear analysis, and sequential analysis. Part III discusses the role of researchers as strategists, and looks into the future of research in human communication disorders.

Advice about how to critically evaluate research, conduct research, and write research reports is given in the appendices.

Examples of research in human communication disorders are given throughout the book. Readers familiar with research methods and statistical analysis can see how the methods and techniques are applied to research in human communication disorders. The aim is to describe the purpose and the function of each aspect of research rather than to give complete technical details; reference is made to texts containing more detailed explanations.

The importance of knowing how to evaluate the strengths and weaknesses of different research approaches is emphasized throughout the book, along with a consideration of strategies for dealing with the practical limitations of research in human communication disorders.

Acknowledgments

I wish to thank Martha Crago, Peter Doehring, Rachel Mayberry, and Eileen Preston for their help with this revised edition.

Introduction

Human communication disorders are difficulties in hearing, speech, and language that impair communication. They occur in both children and adults, and can be present at birth or acquired later in life. The goal of research in human communication disorders is to obtain knowledge that will help persons with communication disorders. There is a reciprocal relationship between research on normal and disordered communication processes. Research on normal communication provides the basis for research on communication disorders, and research on communication disorders can provide important insights concerning normal communication.

For convenience, the abbreviation HCD will be used to denote human communication disorders. The terms *communicative disorders* and *speech, language, and hearing disorders* are also commonly used to describe HCDs.

The quality of HCD research is very high. Competent, imaginative researchers are attracted to this field by the variety of problems that are of vital importance in today's world. Many different kinds of knowledge about HCDs can be useful. An example of the types of useful knowledge that might be obtained about one particular HCD will illustrate this.

AN EXAMPLE OF RESEARCH IN HUMAN COMMUNICATION DISORDERS

Children who make certain errors of omission, distortion, or substitution of speech sounds have communication disorders called *phonological disorders*. A number of different types of research can provide information that is useful in helping children with these disorders.

1

Incidence

Researchers can carry out surveys to determine how frequently phonological disorders occur.

Self-Limiting Nature of Disorders

Developmental research can determine whether some or all children with phonological disorders can outgrow them without any special help.

Assessment

Procedures for reliable assessment of the disorders can be developed through research.

Associated Deficits

Researchers can determine what other deficits might be present in children with these disorders. Deficits that might be associated with phonological disorders include deficiencies in the physical structures (mouth, throat, respiratory system) involved in speech, in the sensory systems (touch, position) involved in speech, in other types of movement (e.g., finger movements), in the perception as well as the production of speech sounds, and in higher level language abilities.

Causes

Research on associated deficits can indicate the extent to which phonological disorders might be the result of structural abnormalities, sensory deficits, general movement disorders, perceptual disorders, or language disorders. Even if no deficits of these types were found, there might be subtle deficiencies in the brain mechanisms that coordinate speech movements. The role played by experience must also be evaluated. Research into the causes of disorders is especially difficult, but can be of basic importance in helping children with these disorders.

Unitary Nature of Disorders

Research concerned with assessment, associated deficits, and possible causes should provide some suggestion as to whether there is a single type of phonological disorder with a single cause. If there does not appear to be a unitary disorder, research can be carried out to determine the number and types of different phonological disorders.

Evaluation of Intervention Methods

Research can be carried out to evaluate intervention methods. If there is not a unitary disorder, different methods may be needed for different types of disorders.

As this example indicates, many kinds of useful knowledge can be obtained by research even when only one specific type of HCD is considered. Much of the research on phonological disorders cited above has already been carried out, but much remains to be done. The exact type of research that will prove useful depends on the type of disorder.

THE USES OF KNOWLEDGE OBTAINED BY RESEARCH

Some knowledge obtained by research can be directly applied. More effective speech intervention procedures and improved hearing aids can be adopted immediately, provided that sufficient confirmation of their benefits has been obtained.

Other knowledge obtained by research can be applied through changes in practice. In the example of phonological disorders, knowledge about the incidence and the self-limiting nature of disorders and about the effectiveness of treatment can help in the planning of programs for dealing with the disorders.

An indirect effect of research is to change theories. Theories concerning phonological disorders that might be changed by research include theories about associated deficits, causes, and different types of disorders, as well as theories about how best to eliminate disorders. Some of these theories can be directly applied to practice, whereas others need to be modified on the basis of further research before they can be applied.

The most indirect effect of research is to suggest further research. Further research can provide additional information about the same problem, or it can lead to a further stage of inquiry. For example, knowledge about deficits associated with phonological disorders might lead to research into the causes of the disorders, and research on causality might lead to research on methods for dealing with the disorders. Research would continue until the knowledge obtained could be applied to theories or practice.

THE NATURE OF KNOWLEDGE OBTAINED BY RESEARCH

HCD research is not aimed at the discovery of absolute truth or universal scientific laws. The knowledge obtained is provisional. The practical needs for dealing with HCDs require that the best current knowledge obtained by research be put to use. The kinds of social and technological processes involved in human communication continue to evolve, creating new research problems.

Provisional knowledge about HCDs is obtained by a variety of research methods. Before the knowledge can be used, it must be evaluated by experts who are familiar with both the methods and the subject matter of the research. A common form of evaluation is the review by experts of research reports submitted for publication in professional journals. This type of *peer evaluation* is the standard procedure for establishing the acceptability of knowledge obtained by research. Because the knowledge is provisional, later research may provide supplementary or contradictory knowledge.

THE NEED FOR KNOWLEDGE OBTAINED BY RESEARCH

Some kinds of knowledge about HCDs are derived from practical experience or theoretical speculation. However, when HCDs are at all complex and variable, research may be necessary to untangle the complexities and account for the sources of variability. Thoughtful, well-planned research is usually the best way to obtain information about such matters as the incidence of disorders, the causes of disorders, the characteristics of disorders, and the effectiveness of treatments. If research has not yet obtained the desired information, then knowledge derived from practical experience and theoretical speculation must be used.

THE CHALLENGE OF HCD RESEARCH

The challenge of HCD research is to make the best use of available methods to obtain useful knowledge. The task is not simple. HCD researchers need patience, dedication, creative ability, and technical expertise, as well as practical experience with HCDs. They determine what knowledge is needed and then try to obtain it as best they can. Difficult though it may be, HCD research offers researchers the opportunity to make important contributions to society. The stakes are high. Practitioners help those particular individuals with whom they work; researchers have the opportunity to obtain information that will help everyone who has an HCD.

RESEARCH STRATEGIES

Researchers use established methods to ensure that their findings will be accepted as valid contributions to knowledge. However, expert researchers, like expert practitioners, do not apply methods mechanically. Each research problem, like each person with an HCD, is unique. Researchers have to adapt available methods to fit each problem. To do so, they must be familiar with current methods and on the lookout for better ones. The term *research strategy* provides an appropriate description of the activities of HCD researchers.

PLAN OF THE BOOK

Following the discussion of research, theory, and practice in this chapter, the different aspects of HCDs studied by researchers are described in Chapter 2. Then the sequence of events in research and the details of designing, carrying out, analyzing, and interpreting research by standard group research methods are given in Part I, which includes Chapters 3 to 14. Review questions and exercises are given at the end of these chapters, where appropriate. Other research methods available to HCD researchers are described in Part II—observational, case study, and descriptive methods in Chapter 15; statistical power analysis, meta-analysis, and multiple methods in Chapter 16; single subject methods in Chapter 17; qualitative methods in Chapter 18; and path analysis, maximum likelihood estimation, loglinear analysis, and sequential analysis in Chapter 19. Part III concerns present and future research strategies in HCD research, with research strategies discussed in Chapter 20 and the future of HCD research discussed in the final chapter. Practical advice about how to read and evaluate research reports, to carry out research, and to prepare research reports is given in three appendices.

Throughout the book there is an emphasis on actual examples of HCD research. The description of standard group research methods in Part I is intended for readers less familiar with research methodology. For readers familiar with these methods, this part will serve as a review and as an indication of how research methods are applied in HCD research. Part II will be of interest to those who wish to learn about other methods that can be used in HCD research.

ADDITIONAL INFORMATION

Additional information about the special nature of HCD research is given in the following books:

Hegde, M. N. (1994). *Clinical research in communicative disorders* (2nd ed.). Austin, TX: PRO-ED.

McReynolds, L. J., & Kearns, K. P. (1983). *Single-subject experimental designs in communicative disorders*. Baltimore: University Park Press.

Shearer, W. M. (1982). *Research processes in speech, language, and hearing*. Baltimore: Williams & Wilkins.

Silverman, F. H. (1977). *Research design in speech pathology and audiology*. Englewood Cliffs, NJ: Prentice-Hall.

Ventry, I. M., & Schiavetti, N. (1980). *Evaluating research in speech pathology and audiology*. New York: Wiley.

◆ ◆ ◆ ◆ ◆ ◆ ◆ REVIEW QUESTIONS ◆ ◆ ◆ ◆ ◆ ◆ ◆

1. Referring to the example of different types of research on articulation/ phonological disorders, describe the kinds of useful knowledge that might be obtained by research on another HCD, such as conductive hearing loss or aphasia.

2. Why is the term *research strategy* used in connection with HCD research?

Aspects of Human Communication Disorders Studied by Researchers

Before the methods and strategies used in HCD research are described, the wide range of problems studied by HCD researchers will be outlined briefly. Anything related to the impairment of face-to-face communication, as well as some other forms of communication, can be studied. Human communication is an ongoing exchange of information between two or more persons. It involves receiving and understanding information, and formulating and expressing responses. During communication, these activities overlap in time. For descriptive purposes, however, it is convenient to consider them as successive stages. HCDs involve difficulty at one or more of these stages of communication.

Receiving communication usually involves listening to speech. Inherited or acquired disorders of peripheral hearing mechanisms may impair listening. The most common peripheral hearing disorders are *conductive* and *sensorineural disorders*. Researchers study the characteristics of these disorders and ways of reducing their effects through hearing aids, operations, cochlear implants, auditory training, and counseling. In cases where listening does not provide enough information, researchers study alternative modes of reception through visual speech cues, sign language, and computer transformation of speech. A great deal of research has been carried out on most aspects of peripheral hearing impairment.

Researchers also study the effects of more central disorders of the neural mechanisms that transmit auditory information to the brain.

These disorders are called *central auditory disorders, auditory perceptual disorders*, and *auditory agnosia*. Much less is known about the characteristics of these disorders and how to help persons who have them.

Inherited and acquired disorders in understanding communicative input can occur at the level of speech sounds, words, sentences, discourse, and communicative intentions (pragmatics). The most common disorders of understanding are *developmental language disorders* in children and *aphasia* in adults. There is a great deal of research concerning the characteristics of these disorders and means of helping persons with them. This research is also useful for theories of normal language development.

Inherited and acquired disorders in formulating and expressing communicative responses involve difficulties in the choice of words, in the articulation of words, and in the vocal quality of speech. The most common disorders are *expressive aphasia, stuttering, phonological disorders, voice disorders*, and expressive disorders associated with cleft palate, cerebral palsy, Parkinson's disease, and laryngectomy. There is a great deal of research on these disorders.

Researchers may concentrate on how a disorder directly affects communication, or on the indirect effects of disorders. For disorders such as stuttering, much of the research is concerned with its direct consequences for communication. For disorders such as early conductive hearing loss and congenital sensorineural hearing impairment, research may focus on how the disorders affect the development of communicative skills. Researchers are also concerned with the effects of HCDs on factors such as personality and school achievement, and on the benefits of intervention.

The scope and diversity of HCD research can be illustrated by listing the titles of research reports in the April 1995 issue of the *Journal of Speech and Hearing Research*:

Dynamic aspects of lower lip movement in Parkinsonian and neurologically normal geriatric speakers' production of stress.

Acoustic prediction of severity in commonly occurring voice problems.

Perceptual rating instrument for speech evaluation in stuttering treatment.

Time-frequency analyses of thyroarytenoid myelectric activity in normal and spasmodic dysphonia patients.

Intelligibility and phonetic contrast errors in highly intelligible speakers with amyotrophic lateral sclerosis.

Identifying the onset and offset of stuttering events.

Acquisition of speech by children who have prolonged cochlear implant experience.

Acoustic correlates of stress in young children's speech.

Effects of lexical meaning and practiced productions on coarticulation in children's and adults' speech.

Effects of linguistic correlates of stuttering on EMG activity in nonstuttering speakers.

Auditory evoked responses to frequency-modulated tones in children with specific language impairment.

Sequential memory in children with and without language impairment.

Phonological working memory and speech production in preschool children.

Measurement of narrative discourse ability in children with language disorders.

Idiom understanding in youth: Further examination of familiarity and transparency.

Quick incidental learning of words by school-age children with and without specific language impairment.

Phonological awareness and literacy development in children with expressive phonological impairments.

Aphasics can distinguish permuted orders of phonemes—But only if presented rapidly.

A study of the tactual reception of sign language.

Confidence limits for maximum word-recognition scores.

Effects of signal and masker uncertainty on children's detection.

HCD research is reported in many other journals, including *Speech, Language, and Hearing Services in the Schools*; *Journal of Speech–Language Pathology and Audiology*; *Journal of Communication Disorders*; and *European Journal of Disorders of Communication*.

Research on specific HCDs is reported in a variety of journals, such as the following:

Hearing disorders—*American Journal of Audiology*; *Audiology*; *Ear and Hearing*; *Journal of Auditory Research*; *Journal of the Acoustical Society of America*; and otolaryngology journals.

Assessment and training of children with hearing impairment—*The Volta Review* and *The American Annals of the Deaf*.

Speech–language disorders—*American Journal of Speech–Language Pathology*.

Developmental language disorders—*Topics in Language Disorders* and linguistic, psycholinguistic, and neurolinguistic journals.

Acquired language disorders—*Aphasiology*; *Brain and Language*; *Neuropsychologia*; and other neuropsychology and neurolinguistics journals.

Stuttering—*Journal of Fluency Disorders*.

Voice disorders—*Journal of Voice* and otolaryngology journals.

Phonological disorders—*Clinical Linguistics and Phonetics*.

Cleft palate—*The Cleft Palate Journal*.

In the past, most HCD researchers were men. This is no longer the case, as indicated by authorship of the 21 research reports in the April 1995 *Journal of Speech and Hearing Research*, where 15 of the first authors were women and 6 were men.

ADDITIONAL INFORMATION

Additional information about aspects of HCDs studied by researchers is best obtained by looking through current issues of the *Journal of Speech and Hearing Research* and the other journals listed above.

✦ ✦ ✦ ✦ ✦ ✦ REVIEW QUESTIONS ✦ ✦ ✦ ✦ ✦ ✦

1. List the stages of human communication and the HCDs at each stage.

2. Take a recent issue of the *Journal of Speech and Hearing Research* and classify each research report according to the stage of communication and the type of HCD studied.

PART I

Standard Group
Research Methods

The chapters in Part I describe standard group research methods that involve probability estimates obtained by statistical analysis of the research data. These methods are used for the vast majority of HCD research. The sequence of events in research, described in Chapter 3, includes the problem, purpose, design, procedure, analysis, and interpretation. Further details concerning research designs are presented in Chapters 4 through 7, procedures in Chapter 8, analysis in Chapters 9 through 13, and interpretation in Chapter 14.

The Sequence of Events in Research

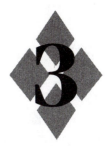

Most HCD research involves a very definite sequence of events. Research is a well-organized exploration. Researchers find a problem that they want to investigate, decide on a specific purpose, design a study to achieve the purpose, collect the data, analyze the data, and interpret the findings. When the research is reported in professional journals, the events are described in their order of occurrence. The research events and the sections of published reports in which they usually appear are shown in Table 3–1.

Each event has its own special importance. The research events are described here in relation to the sections of published research reports in which they appear.

TABLE 3–1. Order of Occurrence of Research Events in Research Reports

RESEARCH EVENTS	RESEARCH REPORTS
Problem (gap in knowledge about HCDs)	Introduction
Purpose (specific aspects to be studied)	Introduction
Design (plan for achieving the purpose)	Introduction or Method
Procedure (operations for carrying out plan)	Method
Analysis (organization of findings)	Results
Interpretation (evaluating findings)	Discussion

PROBLEM

Finding the Problem

Students who are beginning research may learn about a challenging problem from their study of the literature, or from a researcher, teacher, or clinical supervisor. They may become interested in a particular HCD and then look for a gap in knowledge concerning that HCD through reading and consulting experts. Or, they may join a research team that is investigating a particular problem.

Practitioners may become interested in research because they have identified an important gap in knowledge through their clinical work. Then they might seek the collaboration of researchers to plan and carry out research that will reduce the gap.

Experienced researchers often identify a problem through their own previous research. Most gaps in knowledge are not filled by a single study, but require a series of related studies. One of the most important research skills is to decide exactly what problem to investigate at each stage in a series of studies.

Importance of the Problem

Some research contributes small amounts and other research contributes large amounts of knowledge. Everyone is familiar with scientists who stumble on important discoveries by accident. We cannot predict which studies will turn out to be the most important. Both chance and the intuition of the researcher play a part. However, the better informed and more thoughtful the researcher in selecting the problem, the more likely it is to be important.

Specifying the Problem

Once a problem is found, the researcher has to look for previous research and theories that confirm the existence of the gap in knowledge and define it more precisely. This is done by reading relevant books and journals and consulting experts. A great deal of reading and consultation may be needed. The most recent research and theories can be found by reading current issues and consulting annual indexes of relevant journals, writing to leading researchers, and attending research conferences. Computer literature searches are also helpful. Where there has not been a thorough search for previous studies on the topic, the knowledge obtained by research may be of little or no value. There may be repetition of studies that have already been done, or failure to take into consideration important findings of previous researchers.

Statement of the Problem in Research Reports

The gap in knowledge studied by the researcher is described in the first section of the research report. The problem is usually introduced by a discussion of theories and research relating to the gap in knowledge. This defines the general problem area. Then research and theory directly related to the problem are described in more detail, and the gap in knowledge is stated in more specific terms.

The background information and the statement of the problem establish the importance of the research. The editors and reviewers of the journal serve as a jury of peers. They will not accept the research report for publication if they decide that the gap in knowledge has not been adequately defined or the problem is not important. The researcher not only has to find an important problem, but also has to present enough background information within a page or two to demonstrate its importance. Problems are important to the extent that knowledge obtained about them will directly or indirectly benefit persons with HCDs.

Examples of Important Problems

There are many important gaps in knowledge about HCDs, such as the most effective methods for developing language in children with congenital hearing impairment, the exact characteristics of developmental language disorders, and the causes of stuttering and phonological disorders. Such problems are too large to be dealt with by a single research study.

Published studies represent realistic attempts to make progress by obtaining information about selected aspects of important problems. Examples of actual problems studied by HCD researchers are as follows:

1. Do aphasics (adults with acquired language disorders) use non-speech information to help them understand speech? (Records, 1994). (Complete references are given at the end of the chapter).

2. Are older people with hearing loss especially bothered by background noise? (Souza & Turner, 1994).

3. Does language ability affect children's popularity with other children? (Gertner, Rice, & Hadley, 1994).

4. Is improvement in stuttering maintained after treatment is discontinued? (Boberg & Kully, 1994).

In the introductory sections of these research reports, the researchers describe the backgrounds of the problems. The practical importance is not always spelled out, because it is assumed that readers have some previous knowledge of the topic. In the following sections, these four reports will serve as illustrations for the other events described in published research reports.

PURPOSE

After identifying the problem, researchers have to plan a study that will reduce the gap in knowledge. The plan is related to the problem by a statement of the specific purpose of the research. Then a study is designed to accomplish the purpose. Planning continues until a study has been designed that fits the purpose and that is likely to provide acceptable evidence. If a design that will accomplish the purpose cannot be found, the purpose must be modified to fit the available designs.

The Statement of Purpose

The purpose specifies the aspect of the problem that will be investigated. It indicates how much of the gap in knowledge will be reduced and defines the task of research design.

In published HCD research reports, the purpose of the study is usually stated toward the end of the introductory section, sometimes indirectly. The following statements of purpose are taken from the examples of problems in the previous section:

1. "The goal was to obtain information regarding an [aphasic] individual's inclination to make use of visual sources of information when the amount of ambiguity in the speech information was manipulated" (Records, 1994, p. 1087).

2. "The present study was designed to examine the effect of masker modulation in young and elderly listeners" (Souza & Turner, 1994, p. 659).

3. "In this study, the relationship between linguistic competence and social status was examined for three groups of children enrolled in a mainstreamed preschool classroom" (Gertner et al., 1994, p. 915).

4. "The purpose of this paper is to report on an investigation of the long-term effects of an intensive group program for adult and adolescent stutterers" (Boberg & Kully, 1994, p. 1051).

DESIGN

Researchers have to plan studies that will provide the information specified by the statement of purpose. Such planning involves the selection of an appropriate research design, a number of which are available for use. To plan, understand, and evaluate HCD research, it is necessary to be familiar with the most commonly used designs. Research designs are briefly described here to indicate their function in the sequence of research events. A detailed description of standard group research designs is given in Chapters 5 and 6.

The most common designs obtain information about one or more groups, using methods developed for psychological research. Information about the characteristics of HCDs can be obtained by comparing groups with HCDs to groups without HCDs, by comparing groups with different types of HCDs, or by analyzing relevant characteristics of a single group. Information about the effectiveness of methods for helping persons with HCDs can be obtained by assessing groups with HCDs before and after the methods have been applied.

Description of Research Designs in Published Reports

Research designs are often described briefly at the end of the introductory section of published research reports, with further details of the design given in the second section, Method. The description of the design may also be given in a subsection called Design, but is more often combined with the description of the procedure. The design must provide an acceptable means of achieving the stated purpose. The designs for the four published research reports used here for illustration can be summarized as follows:

1. The comprehension of aphasics with good and poor language comprehension was assessed in situations involving speech alone, gestures alone, and speech plus gestures, where the speech and gestural information varied in ambiguity (Records, 1994).

2. The speech recognition of young and elderly listeners with hearing loss was assessed under four conditions of background noise varying in their speechlike nature (Souza & Turner, 1994).

3. Popularity with peers was assessed in preschool children with normally developing language, with speech and/or language impairment, and with English as a second language (Gertner et al., 1994).

4. Speech fluency of adolescent and adult stutterers was assessed before, during, and after an intensive treatment program (Boberg & Kully, 1994).

PROCEDURE

The research design is an abstract description of the study. To put the design into practice, two further stages of planning are necessary. Decisions must be made about the exact procedure necessary to fulfill the requirements of the design. Then the researchers must determine whether resources are available to carry out the procedure. If not, the procedure and perhaps the design must be modified to fit the available resources. If this cannot be done, the study may have to be abandoned. Procedures used in HCD research are briefly described here, with more details given in Chapter 8.

Deciding on the Procedure

When the design has been made, it is necessary to decide exactly what subjects will be studied, what characteristics of the subjects will be assessed, and how the assessments will be carried out. This aspect of research is just as important as the problem, the purpose, and the design of the study. The subjects have to be representative of the populations being studied, the characteristics assessed have to provide valid and reliable information about the processes studied, and the assessments have to be obtained in a well-controlled manner that rules out the possible influence of extraneous factors.

Determining Available Resources

The decisions concerning the procedure can be put into action only if the required resources are available. These include subjects with HCDs and subjects without HCDs, equipment and materials, facilities for assessment or training, and research personnel. The research personnel (often the researchers themselves) must be able to operate the equipment, make measurements, administer testing and training procedures required by the research, and analyze the results.

When the required resources are not available, the procedure must be modified, or an attempt must be made to obtain them. For the types of research that are published as useful contributions to knowledge about HCDs, the necessary resources are often obtained by means of research grants from government agencies or private foundations.

Description of the Procedure in Published Reports

The procedure is described in the Method section of published research reports. Enough details should be given so that someone else could repeat the study. As stated above, the description of the procedure is often combined with the description of the design.

The subjects are usually described in a subsection entitled Subjects. Equipment and materials are described in subsections with headings such as Tasks, Apparatus, Tests, Measures, and Instrumentation. The operations for obtaining the required information about subjects are described in subsections with headings such as Procedure, Test Procedure, or Training Procedure.

The procedures of the four illustrative research reports are summarized as follows:

1. Seven aphasic subjects with high comprehension and five aphasic subjects with low comprehension pointed to one of two pictures in response to an audiotaped sentence, a videotaped gesture, or both. The sentence and the gesture varied in ambiguity (Records, 1994).

2. Ten young adult and ten elderly listeners with mild-to-moderate sensorineural hearing loss, and ten young adult listeners with normal hearing repeated lists of 50 spoken monosyllabic words under conditions of high-pass noise, speech-spectrum noise plus high-pass noise, babble-modulated noise plus high-pass noise, and babble plus high-pass noise (Souza & Turner, 1994).

3. Nine children with normal language development, twelve children with speech and/or language impairment, and ten children whose second language was English, all 4 to 5 years old and all in the same preschool classroom, were asked to point to pictures of children they liked to play with and children they did not like to play with, and were also given a picture vocabulary test (Gertner et al., 1994).

4. Seventeen adult stutterers and twenty-five adolescent stutterers completed a 3-week intensive stuttering program. Speech samples were obtained immediately before and after treatment, and 4, 12, and 24 months after treatment. A speech performance questionnaire was sent to subjects 12 to 24 months after treatment (Boberg & Kully, 1994).

ANALYSIS

Data analysis is another essential research event. Even when resources are available for collecting the data, the researchers have to find appropriate methods for analyzing it, and must have the resources for carrying out the analysis, which can be very complex and time-consuming. If there are difficulties, fewer subjects may be studied or fewer measures obtained per subject. Data analyses can be greatly facilitated by microcomputer programs.

Decisions about data analysis should be made at the same time as decisions about the design. The design may have to be changed if appropriate techniques of analysis are not available. Several different types of data analysis are possible. The type of analysis most appropriate for a particular study will depend on the purpose, the design, and the available procedures.

Before the information obtained in a study can be analyzed, it may be necessary to put the data into a different form. This stage of data analysis is called *data reduction*. Then the analysis itself may involve numerical descriptions, statements of probability derived from statistical tests, or written descriptions. The different stages of analysis are briefly described here and are described in more detail in Chapters 9 to 13.

Data Reduction

After the desired information has been collected in the manner pre-scribed by the procedure, it must be expressed in a way that is inter-pretable as evidence regarding the problem. Sometimes the information can be used in its original form; for example, the effects of a drug that causes hearing loss might be demonstrated by showing audiograms of several patients before and after administration of the drug. In most studies, however, one or more stages of data reduction is required.

When information about communication has been recorded on audio-tape or videotape, the data have to be transcribed into written form. This is a very time-consuming process, and resources may be available only for transcription of a restricted sample of the information. Judgments that put the transcribed responses into categories may be necessary for further analysis. This usually requires experienced judges and may be a lengthy process. It is often necessary to demonstrate the reliability of the tran-scriptions and the categorical judgments by statistical procedures that compare the transcriptions or judgments of two or more persons.

Descriptive Statistics

Descriptive statistics are measures that organize data to give detailed information for individuals and that summarize data to show measures of average performance and variability for groups. Interpretations can be directly based on this descriptive information. Descriptive statistics are used in almost all research reports, often as a supplement to inferential statistics. The detailed information provided by descriptive statistics can often be directly related to the concerns of practitioners.

Inferential Statistics

The numerical information in descriptive statistics can be further ana-lyzed by inferential statistics to arrive at estimates of the probability that the observed effects would be found in other subjects of the same type. Statistical tests are used in group studies to assess differences between two or more groups, to assess change in one or more groups, and to determine the degree of relationship between selected characteristics of a group.

Statistical tests require mathematical calculations of varying degrees of complexity. At one time, the lengthy calculations required by complex statistics made it impossible to carry out many studies, but microcomputer statistical programs have made even the most lengthy and complex analyses available to most researchers.

Description of Data Analyses in Published Reports

In published research reports, the techniques used for data analysis are often described in the Method section, sometimes in a subsection entitled Data Analysis. The results of the data analysis are presented in the Results section. Descriptive and inferential statistics are usually presented in tables and graphs. Qualitative analyses are presented as written descriptions.

The data analyses for the four illustrative research reports can be summarized as follows:

1. Descriptive statistics (graphs of individual and group results) and inferential statistics (repeated measures analyses and t-tests) were used in the study of gesture and speech perception in aphasics (Records, 1994).

2. Descriptive statistics (means and standard deviations of group results) and inferential statistics (analysis of variance and analysis of covariance with post hoc tests) were used in the study of background noise, age, and hearing loss (Souza & Turner, 1994).

3. Descriptive statistics (means and standard deviations of group results and individual standard scores) and inferential statistics (analysis of variance with post hoc tests and correlation tests) were used in the study of language ability and popularity in preschool children (Gertner et al., 1994).

4. Descriptive statistics (individual results and group means) were used in the study of long-term results of a stuttering treatment program (Boberg & Kully, 1994).

INTERPRETATION

After the data collected by researchers have been analyzed, the information provided by the analysis is evaluated in relation to the purpose of the study. Then the findings are related to the original problem, and conclusions are reached about the new information contributed by the research.

Only rarely does the new information completely close the gap in practical knowledge that suggested the problem.

The interpretation can serve several very important functions. Conclusions may be reached regarding the extent to which the findings apply to others with HCDs, the implications of the findings for direct practical applications may be stated, and suggestions can be made for further research. More details regarding interpretation are given in Chapter 14.

In published research reports, the interpretation is given in sections called Discussion, Results and Discussion, or Discussion and Conclusions, which usually provide detailed descriptions of how the results relate to the problem and to previous research. The conclusions usually state the contribution of the findings to theoretical and practical knowledge, and are sometimes given in a separate section entitled Conclusions or Implications.

Interpretations of the four illustrative research reports can be summarized as follows:

1. As auditory information becomes more ambiguous, aphasics with comprehension deficits make greater use of gestural information (Records, 1994).

2. The effects of speechlike background noise were not significantly different for young normal listeners, young listeners with hearing loss, and elderly listeners with hearing loss (Souza & Turner, 1994).

3. Children with normal language development tended to be preferred by their peers; children with language impairment and children learning English as a second language tended to receive negative peer nominations (Gertner et al., 1994).

4. Over two thirds of the stutterers maintained a satisfactory level of posttreatment fluency (Boberg & Kully, 1994).

STRATEGIES

HCD research is seldom carried out under ideal circumstances. Previous research and theory rarely provide an exact definition of the gap in knowledge. Available research designs and methods of data analysis cannot always provide information directly applicable to HCDs. Subjects, materials, and facilities may not be available to meet the requirements of the research design and data analyses. Such limitations prevent researchers from obtaining all the information they need in one study. The findings may only suggest the kind of further research that should be done.

Under these circumstances, HCD researchers cannot simply be well-trained methodologists who apply a fixed set of techniques to achieve certain knowledge. They must be strategists who go as far as they can toward achieving their practical goals by whatever means are available. Somewhat different skills are required for each of the research events. Creativity, intuition, and practical knowledge are needed to identify an important problem, scholarship to search out previous theories and research, technical knowledge to make the plan and analyze the data, resourcefulness and diligent attention to detail to carry out the procedure, and interpretive abilities to explain the contribution to knowledge.

In addition to these separate skills, researchers have to integrate the research events. The purpose has to fit the problem and the design; the design has to fit the purpose, the procedure, and the data analysis; the procedure has to fit the design and the available resources; and the data analysis has to fit the design, procedure, and purpose. To accomplish this integration, researchers have to be well informed, adaptable, ingenious, and highly goal oriented.

The skills needed for HCD research are not completely different from those needed for practice. Like professional practice, research requires knowledge, skill, and determination.

Description of Research Strategies in Published Reports

The published studies of successful HCD researchers show how research strategies are employed to achieve the practical goals of HCD research. In the four examples used here, the strategies can be summarized as follows:

1. A method for assessing the use of gestural information in speech comprehension adapted from other investigators was validated with subjects with normal hearing. Both individual and group results were obtained for two groups of aphasics (Records, 1994).

2. Different kinds of speechlike background noise were used to simulate noisy listening conditions for young and elderly listeners with hearing loss (Souza & Turner, 1994).

3. A procedure adapted from other investigators was used to determine which classmates children liked to play with and which
classmates they did not like to play with. The effects of language
development on peer preference were determined by comparing
normally developing children with children who had language
impairments and children who were learning English as a second
language, all in the same classroom (Gertner et al., 1994).

4. Speech samples obtained via the telephone and questionnaire
responses were used to assess the effects of an intensive stuttering
treatment program; interpretations were based on descriptive statistics only (Boberg & Kully, 1994).

In all four examples, the researchers obtained quantifiable information
that was intended to estimate the effects of HCDs in a real-life situation.
A major challenge of HCD research strategists is to figure out ways to
obtain evidence of this sort. No single strategy will suit all the different
problems of HCD research.

ADDITIONAL INFORMATION

Additional information regarding the sequence of research events is given
in the books on HCD research listed at the end of Chapter 1, and in texts
on psychological research methods, such as those listed at the end of the
next chapter.

References

Boberg, E., & Kully, D. (1994). Long-term results of an intensive treatment program for adults and adolescents who stutter. *Journal of Speech and Hearing
Research, 37*, 1050–1059.

Gertner, B. L., Rice, M. L., & Hadley, P. A. (1994). Influence of communicative
competence on peer preferences in a preschool classroom. *Journal of Speech
and Hearing Research, 37*, 913–923.

Records, N. L. (1994). A measure of the contribution of a gesture to the perception of speech in listeners with aphasia. *Journal of Speech and Hearing
Research, 37*, 1086–1099.

Souza, P. E., & Turner, C. W. (1994). Masking of speech in young and elderly listeners with hearing loss. *Journal of Speech and Hearing Research, 37,* 655–661.

❖ ❖ ❖ ❖ ❖ ❖ ❖ **REVIEW QUESTIONS** ❖ ❖ ❖ ❖ ❖ ❖ ❖

1. List the sequence of events in research, briefly describe each event, and indicate where they are described in research reports.

2. Find the research events in all of the research reports in a recent issue of the *Journal of Speech and Hearing Research.*

Basic Principles of Research Design

To select an important problem, researchers must know about HCDs and be aware of gaps in knowledge. Then a study is designed to accomplish a specific purpose related to the problem. Special knowledge about designs applicable to HCD research is required. This technical knowledge is a basic tool of HCD research.

The problems investigated by HCD research require a variety of designs. The types of design traditionally used by HCD researchers are described in Chapters 5 and 6. These designs permit statistical analysis of differences between and within groups of subjects. Underlying the designs are certain basic principles of research design. These principles are discussed in the present chapter.

CONTROLS

Theorists increase our understanding of HCDs by creative integration of present knowledge. Researchers obtain new knowledge about HCDs by observation. Research designs provide the rules for observation. The rules for observation of parent–child communication in natural settings are quite different from the rules for laboratory observation of very restricted aspects of ear drum or tongue movement. A detailed explanation of *controls* and *variables* is essential to an understanding of the basic principles or rules of research design.

A control is a restriction of natural variation. Research designs control natural variations to isolate the variables that are to be studied. The variables that are controlled in HCD research include characteristics of the subjects who participate in the research and characteristics of the situation in which the observations are made. Control of the subject and situational variables permits researchers to study the effects of the variables in which they are interested.

The extent to which each kind of variation is controlled depends on the research design. Because HCD research is designed to achieve practical goals, complete control of all variables of possible interest is seldom if ever achieved. As a result, HCD researchers must be extremely cautious in interpreting their findings. An important aspect of interpretation is to evaluate the extent to which all relevant variables have been controlled.

Subject Controls

The type of HCD to be studied is controlled by the selection of subjects who have that type of HCD. To isolate the effects of the HCD, subjects of a certain age, gender, cultural background, education, and history of treatment may be studied. In such a case, these subject variables are controlled by holding them constant. If these variables were not controlled, attempts to study the effects of the HCD might be confounded by the effects of the uncontrolled variables.

Another control procedure is to compare subjects with HCDs to subjects without HCDs. The control subjects are commonly formed into groups called control groups. The control group is matched with a group of HCD subjects on variables such as age, gender, and cultural background. To the extent that the groups can be matched on relevant variables, the effects of the HCD will be isolated. To the extent that all relevant variables are not controlled, the effects of the HCD are not completely isolated.

Not all HCD research involves the comparison of HCD groups and control groups. Some designs compare only groups of HCD subjects differing in type of HCD, age, gender, history of treatment, or other variables. Relevant variables are also controlled in the selection of such groups. Other designs involve repeated measurements of a single group. The controls required for such designs will be discussed later. Still other designs study individuals rather than groups. In such designs, the interpretation of differences between individuals depends on the extent to which relevant variables have been controlled.

Situation Controls

In addition to controlling subject variables, the research design controls the situation. If the variable studied is the detection of sounds, for instance, sounds will be presented under carefully controlled acoustic conditions in which background noise and reverberation are kept to a minimum to isolate the effect of the experimental sound. If the variable studied is stuttering, the speech situation may be controlled by the use of a standardized interview to reduce the possibility that the amount and type of stuttering are influenced by situational variability.

Other situational variables may also be controlled. If an observer is present who records observations, controls may be necessary to rule out the possibility that the observer's expectations will affect the observations. Likewise, it may be necessary to carefully word the instructions to subjects in order to control the possibility that their expectations will affect their performance.

The need for situational controls varies with the type of design. For example, researchers who wish to determine how sounds are detected in real-life situations will not control background noise and reverberation. Similarly, researchers who wish to assess stuttering in natural situations will not restrict observations to carefully controlled speaking situations. Even in natural situations, however, some control needs to be exerted. HCD researchers studying communication in natural settings would usually observe only situations in which communication is likely to occur, and perhaps would exert some control over the situation. The caregiver may be asked to play with the child who is being observed so that a particularly important form of natural communication may be observed.

The Importance of Controls

Controls are essential for achieving the purposes of standard group research. If the variables under study are not isolated by controlling relevant variables, alternative explanations of the findings cannot be ruled out. For example, to determine whether children with language disorders are deficient in speech–sound perception, it is necessary to rule out the possibilities that observed differences in speech perception are not a function of age, gender, linguistic background, hearing impairment, the acoustic and linguistic characteristics of the speech sounds, the listening conditions, or the expectations of the subjects or observers.

Decisions regarding which variables to control are extremely important. If necessary controls have not been applied, the purpose of research may not be accomplished. A study in which relevant variables have not been controlled is seriously flawed, and reports may yield very misleading information about HCDs.

VARIABLES

Control and variability represent the opposite extremes of order and disorder. Both are essential to research. In carefully controlled studies, subject and situation variables are controlled. Only the phenomena of interest are allowed to vary. The variables that have been described above as "phenomena of interest," "experimental treatments," and "the variable under study" are those whose effects are isolated by controlling relevant variables. The technical term for these variables is *independent variable*. The technical term for the observed effects of varying the independent variables is *dependent variable*. To understand how research designs work, it is necessary to understand these terms fully.

Independent Variables

Terminology concerning controls and variables can be confusing. Researchers systematically vary the independent variable by controlling its variation. The research design is described in terms of the systematic variation of the independent variables, the observation of the effects of the independent variables on the dependent variables, and the systematic control of other variables that might produce variation in the dependent variables. Researchers vary independent variables to observe their effects on dependent variables. Through all of these descriptions runs the idea that independent variables provide the information that fills gaps in knowledge about HCDs.

The aspect of the independent variable that is varied by the research design is the *level* of the independent variable. The levels can involve quantitative or qualitative variations. Quantitative variations could be different age levels, or different levels of background masking noise.

Qualitative variations could be subjects of different genders or different types of communication situation. The effects of two or more levels of an independent variable and of two or more independent variables can be studied. In this way, complex, multidimensional information about HCDs can be obtained by a single experimental design.

Like control variables, independent variables can be subject variables or situation variables. Examples of independent subject variables are HCD versus non-HCD, intervention versus no intervention, type of intervention, type of HCD, age, gender, cultural background, and history of intervention. Examples of independent situation variables are sound frequency, masking noise, and different communication situations. All such variables can either be held constant as controlled variables or systematically varied as independent variables, depending on the purpose of the research.

Dependent Variables

After designing research as best they can, researchers observe what happens. The outcome of the controls and variations dictated by research designs is variation in the dependent variables. Variations in dependent variables are recorded by *quantitative* or *qualitative* observations. In studies of voice disorders, the dependent variables might be quantitative acoustic measures or qualitative perceptual judgments of hoarseness or breathiness. In research on hearing, the dependent variables might be quantitative measures of hearing thresholds at different frequencies or qualitative judgments by subjects with hearing impairments of their feelings about being hearing impaired. In research on language disorders, the dependent variables might be quantitative judgments of the syntactic complexity of written stories or qualitative descriptions of communicative interactions.

The data provided by dependent variables are evaluated and interpreted to determine how much knowledge about HCDs has been obtained. The degree of confidence that can be placed in the findings depends in part on how well the design has controlled relevant variables and isolated the effects of independent variables. It also depends on the extent to which the design is appropriate to the problem, and on the repeatability of the observations. The design is evaluated in terms of *validity* and the observations are evaluated in terms of *reliability*. These are the two remaining principles of research design to be considered in this chapter.

VALIDITY AND RELIABILITY

The independent and dependent variables in an experimental design are carefully selected to achieve new knowledge. The knowledge will be most helpful if the measure of the dependent variable is both reliable and valid. A measure is valid to the extent that it measures what it claims to measure, and reliable to the extent that it is consistent and repeatable.

Validity

The two kinds of validity that are most important for HCD research are *internal validity* and *external validity*. A study is internally valid when relevant variables have been controlled, and the only variables that affect the dependent variables are the independent variables. When uncontrolled variables can affect the dependent variable, the effects of the independent variable are *confounded* with the effects of the uncontrolled variables. For example, if the effects of age and other relevant variables are not controlled, a study of the effects of lipreading training on communicative competence may be confounded. The success of standard research designs depends on the control of variables that might confound the effects of the independent variables.

External validity is the extent to which the effects of independent variables on dependent variables in the research situation apply to the natural setting. How does the ability of children who are hearing impaired to repeat isolated words relate to the intelligibility of their speech in natural settings? If the information obtained by research does not have external validity, it may not be of immediate practical use. The term *ecological validity* is sometimes used in addition to the term external validity to describe the need for experimental findings to apply to natural settings.

Reliability

Measurements of dependent variables are reliable to the extent that the same measurements would be obtained if the study were repeated. If the measures are numerical scores, it may be important to estimate how much the scores would vary if the test were repeated. If the measurements are judgments by an observer, it may be necessary to determine whether other observers would make the same judgments. Any source of inconsistency that produces variation in the measurement of the independent variables may confound the effects of the independent variables. The reliability of measurements can be estimated in several ways. *Test–retest reliability* is assessed by obtaining the same measure twice and comparing the two measures. *Split-half reliability* can be assessed when measurements consist of a series of items. The items are split in half and the resulting measurements compared. *Alternate form reliability* can be assessed when alternative forms of measurement are compared. *Observer reliability* is assessed when the judgments of two or more observers are compared.

Both reliability and validity must be taken into consideration in designing and interpreting experiments that are intended to provide useful information about HCDs.

BASIC PRINCIPLES OF HCD RESEARCH

One of the most crucial aspects of HCD research is the careful selection of the variables that are to be controlled or systematically varied. After a problem has been found and the purpose specified, there must be a consideration of which variables are most relevant to the problem and the purpose. HCDs are complex, and the relevant variables are not always obvious. If relevant variables are not taken into consideration, practical applications of the research findings may have negative consequences for persons with HCDs.

Most HCD research designs do not just involve one independent variable, one dependent variable, and a small set of controlled variables. Rather than holding age and gender constant in studying the language skills of children who are hearing impaired, researchers may wish to determine the effects of age and gender on language skill by systematically varying them. Likewise, researchers may not obtain sufficient information to achieve the purpose of assessing the language skills of children who are hearing impaired by observing only one type of language skill, but may wish to observe the effects of hearing impairment on vocabulary, grammar, and connected discourse.

The purpose of the research governs the selection of the independent and dependent variables. The research design prescribes reliable observations that will lead to valid conclusions concerning the effects of the independent variables on the dependent variables. A clear understanding of the functions of controls and variables and the concepts of reliability and validity is the key to understanding the basic principles of research design.

The amount and type of control and variation and the need to demonstrate reliability and validity depend on the aspects of HCDs studied and the purpose of the research. Researchers must familiarize themselves with the different kinds of research designs in order to select those most appropriate for the problems they wish to study. The function of controls and variables in research designs is most easily illustrated in simple group research designs borrowed from psychological research, as described in the next chapter.

ADDITIONAL INFORMATION

Basic principles of research design are discussed in texts on research methods, such as the following:

Adams, G. R., & Schvaneveldt, J. D. (1991). *Understanding research methods* (2nd ed.). White Plains, NY: Longman.

Graziano, A. M., & Raulin, M. L. (1993). *Research methods: A process of inquiry* (2nd ed.). New York: HarperCollins.

Shaughnessy, J. J., & Zechmeister, E. B. (1985). *Research methods in psychology.* New York: Knopf.

❖ ❖ ❖ ❖ ❖ ❖ ❖ **REVIEW QUESTION** ❖ ❖ ❖ ❖ ❖ ❖ ❖

Briefly define the following terms: *controls, variables, subject controls, situation controls, confounding, relevant variables, independent variables, levels of independent variables, dependent variables, validity, reliability, internal validity, external validity, test–retest reliability, split-half reliability, alternate form reliability,* and *observer reliability.*

❖ ❖ ❖ ❖ ❖ ❖ ❖ ❖ ❖ **EXERCISES** ❖ ❖ ❖ ❖ ❖ ❖ ❖ ❖ ❖

(answers are given in Appendix D)

1. Researchers wish to find out if children with speech production disorders also have difficulty understanding speech. They give a speech

perception test to a group of children with phonological disorders and a group of children without phonological disorders. The test consists of 50 items, each of which requires the child to point to one of three pictures that represent a spoken word.

a. List relevant subject and situation controls.

b. Give an example of the confounding of the effects of articulation disorders by an uncontrolled variable.

c. What are the independent and the dependent variables?

d. What are the levels of the independent variable?

e. How would internal validity and external validity be determined?

f. How could the reliability of the speech perception test be determined?

g. Would it be necessary to assess observer reliability? (Explain.)

2. Researchers wish to evaluate a new treatment for stuttering. They record a speech sample from a group of stutterers before and after training.

a. What are the independent and dependent variables?

b. What are the levels of the independent variable?

c. How would external validity be determined?

d. Should reliability be assessed? (Say what type and how.)

3. Researchers wish to evaluate a new treatment for stuttering. They record speech samples from a group of stutterers who have been given a new type of training and a group of stutterers who have not been given the new type of training.

a. What are the independent and dependent variables?

b. What are the levels of the independent variable?

c. List relevant subject and situation controls.

d. Which group is the control group?

e. Give an example of the confounding of the effects of training by an uncontrolled variable.

Simple Group
Research Designs

Group research designs isolate the effects of independent variables by controlling for the inherent variability of human behavior. Behavior is much more variable than physiological processes. The operation of the circulatory, respiratory, and digestive systems is more uniform in all persons. Physiologists record responses that do not vary greatly from one person to another under standard laboratory conditions. As a result, they can obtain knowledge of human physiology by carefully controlled observations of a small number of individuals.

Human behavior varies greatly as a function of a host of variables, including age, gender, personality, education, culture, and individual life experience. Even under the most standard laboratory conditions, there will be individual differences in the behaviors studied. Researchers attempt to overcome this variability by estimating the probability that one set of carefully controlled observations is different from another set of carefully controlled observations.

Research concerned with the physiological aspects of HCDs does not usually require standard group research designs. A great deal of HCD research does, however, involve the kind of variable behavior for which group designs were developed. Even then, group designs may not be appropriate. Information about groups is not always suitable to the practical purposes of HCD research.

Simple group designs are described in this chapter. Complex group designs are described in the next chapter. The advantages and disadvantages of traditional group research designs for HCD research are discussed in Chapter 7.

The simplest group designs involve one independent variable with two levels, and one dependent variable. The levels of the independent variable can be independent groups or repeated measurements. These two types of design will be discussed separately.

INDEPENDENT GROUP DESIGNS

In simple independent group designs, the independent variable has two levels, represented by two independent groups. There are four types of independent group designs—random selection, random assignment, matched group, and natural group designs. The natural group design is most commonly used in HCD research.

Random Selection Designs

The basic design is the random selection design for two groups. The groups are randomly selected from the same population. There is one independent variable with two levels, and one dependent variable. One group receives one level of the independent variable and the other group receives the other level. The effect of varying the independent variable is indicated by the difference between groups on the dependent variable.

Variables such as age, gender, and education are controlled by random selection of subjects, which insures that there will be no systematic differences between groups for these variables. Situation variables are held as constant as possible for all subjects in both groups. When these simple rules of research design have been followed, a statistical analysis can be carried out to estimate the probability that the value of the dependent variable for Group 1 differs from that for Group 2, thus accomplishing the purpose of the research.

For example, two groups of 100 children are randomly selected from the total population of children with language disorders. The independent variable is vocabulary training. One group is given extensive training in which new words are introduced in the context of stories and the other group is given no training. Then both groups take a vocabulary test that includes the new words. The score on the vocabulary test is the dependent variable. Subject variables such as age, gender, and education are controlled by allowing them to vary randomly. Situation variables such as testing room, time of testing, and the person giving the vocabulary test are held constant. The difference between groups in vocabulary test scores is evaluated by statistical analysis to estimate the effect of training in defining words on the vocabularies of children with language disorders.

This standard design is described by standard terms. The *independent variable* is the *treatment*. The two *levels* of the treatment are vocabulary training and no vocabulary training. The group receiving the treatment is the *experimental group* and the group receiving no treatment is the *control group*. The term *control* is also applied to situational variables that are held constant for both groups. The measure of the effect of the treatment (vocabulary test score) is the *dependent variable*.

A group research design was used to study the effects of vocabulary training. Vocabulary is a variable psychological process. With the simple random group design, the independent variable was isolated by a random selection procedure that controlled subject variables. Careful control of the experimental situation ensured that relevant variables other than the independent variable were held constant. Then the effect of the independent variable could be demonstrated by differences between groups on the dependent variable.

If the rules of this simple design are followed, researchers can evaluate the effects of training in a rigorous, scientifically acceptable manner. Such a design could be very useful for HCD research. However, random selection from an entire population, with or without HCDs, is virtually impossible for HCD researchers. Even if it were not, many researchers would prefer to systematically control variables such as age, gender, and education rather than allowing them to vary randomly.

Random Assignment Designs

Random assignment designs overcome the difficulty of access to an entire population. When only a restricted population of subjects is available, they can be randomly assigned to one group or the other. Like the random selection procedure, subject variables are controlled by allowing them to vary randomly. Except for the population from which subjects are selected, there is no difference between random selection and random assignment designs. All of the other characteristics of random selection designs apply to random assignment designs.

Random assignment designs are more feasible than random selection designs for HCD research. The researcher can randomly assign two groups from whatever population is available. However, the design has potential drawbacks. The restricted population from which the subjects are selected may not be representative of the entire population. For example, a group of children with language disorders from one city may differ in cultural and linguistic background from the entire population of children with language disorders. In such a case, the research findings would apply only to language disorders with the characteristics of that particular population.

Another potential difficulty with random assignment designs is that the relatively small populations available for random selection may be extremely variable. Subjects may differ greatly in relevant subject variables. In such cases, the dependent variable might vary a great deal as a function of these subject variables. The variability within groups and between groups might obscure the effect of the independent variable. For example, randomly assigned groups of children with language disorders might vary greatly in vocabulary as a function of age, education, cultural background, and language background. Such variation might be quite large relative to the variation resulting from the vocabulary training of one group.

Matched Group Designs

The subject variability that may be a problem in random assignment designs can be overcome by matched group designs. In the simple matched group design, one or more variables that may affect the dependent variable can be held constant between groups by matching the groups on those variables. There are two types of matched group design. In treatment studies, the two groups can be matched on the dependent variable prior to treatment. They are selected in such a way that both groups have the same average score on the dependent variable. For example, in a vocabulary training study, the two groups can be matched on the basis of a vocabulary test given prior to training. Then, any differences between groups in vocabulary after training can be attributed to the independent variable, training versus nontraining.

In the other type of matched group design, groups are matched on variables other than the dependent variable. Variables are selected for matching that might affect the dependent variable, such as age, gender, and education. This matching procedure, like the pretreatment matching procedure described above, should help to isolate the effects of the independent variable. Differences between groups matched on relevant variables should reflect the effects of the independent variable. If two groups could not be matched in vocabulary prior to training, they could be matched in age, gender, education, and cultural background to control the effects of these variables on the dependent variable. Then any differences between groups in vocabulary could be more clearly attributed to the independent variable of training.

The final consideration for matched group designs is the exact form of matching. If two groups are to be matched in vocabulary, the minimum requirement is that both groups have the same average vocabulary prior to training. Variability in pretraining vocabulary can be reduced even further if the distribution of vocabulary scores around the mean (group average) is the same for both groups. Then the more restricted the distribution, the better will be the control of pretraining vocabulary. The effects of vocabulary training are more easily demonstrated for groups whose pretraining vocabularies vary within a very limited range.

The same reasoning holds true for matching on other variables. Not only the average age, but also the distribution of ages of the two groups should be the same, and the best control of age is for both groups to be at a single age level. This is most important in studies of infants and young children, for whom developmental changes are large. Both groups should have the same proportion of boys and girls, and gender effects are best controlled if all subjects are of the same gender. Similarly, education and cultural background are best controlled if all subjects are at the same educational level and come from the same cultural background. These restrictions in the range of variation of matched variables will enhance the observed effects of the independent variable.

The matched group design is very appropriate for HCD research, because the relatively small populations available to most researchers make it very difficult to select comparable groups by random assignment. In matched group designs, like random selection and random assignment designs, the independent and dependent variable are clearly defined and other variables that may affect the dependent variable are controlled. What is sacrificed in the simple matched group design as compared with the random selection design is the ability to generalize the findings to the entire population. If all subjects are of the same age, gender, education, and cultural background, the findings may not apply to subjects of other ages, genders, educational levels, and cultural backgrounds. Designs that help to overcome problems of restricted generality are discussed in the next chapter.

Natural Group Designs

The remaining type of simple independent group design is the natural group design. In this design, the groups are selected from two different populations. The designs previously discussed select two groups from the same population, and the independent variable is different treatment of the two groups. In the natural group design, the independent variable is a difference between groups "created by nature" that exists prior to the selection of the groups. The effect of this independent variable is studied. Other variables that might affect the dependent variable are controlled by random selection or by matching.

For example, a randomly selected group of boys can be compared with a randomly selected group of girls in their performance on a vocabulary test to determine whether girls have better vocabularies than boys. The independent variable is gender, the dependent variable is once again vocabulary score, and all other variables are uncontrolled.

An important limitation of natural group designs is that the groups may differ in subtle ways that are not easy to detect or to control. Differences between groups may be attributable to these uncontrolled variables rather than to the independent variable. In the comparison of girls and boys, for example, differences in vocabulary might be attributable to different cultural attitudes toward girls and boys rather than to natural (that is, biological) differences.

Combined Natural Group and Matched Group Designs

A design commonly used in HCD research is the combined matched group and natural group design. The restricted samples of HCD subjects available to researchers usually rule out random selection and assignment, making it necessary to match groups on relevant variables. In studies in which HCD groups are compared with normal control groups, the natural group design must be used, because the two groups come from different populations. This is also true of comparisons between HCD groups that differ in type or severity of HCD, or in other variables such as age and gender. Since the combined matched group and natural group design is so important for HCD research, several examples will be given.

It may be important to determine whether children with phonological disorders also have higher level language disorders. Higher level language skills of a natural group of children with phonological disorders and a natural group of children without phonological disorders would be compared. The independent variable would be the presence of phonological disorders. The dependent variable would be a measure of higher level language skill (for example, a vocabulary test or a grammar test). A restricted group of children with phonological disorders would be available. The control group of children without phonological disorders would be selected to match the phonological disorder group in relevant variables such as age, gender, education, and cultural background.

If all relevant variables had been controlled, a difference between groups on the measure of higher level language skill would provide evidence that children with phonological disorders do have higher level language disorders. However, the difference might be attributable to variables other than phonology per se, such as organic or environmental factors associated with phonological disorders. It could not, therefore, be concluded that there is a cause-and-effect relationship between phonological disorders and higher level language disorders. All that could be concluded is that children with phonological disorders tend to have higher level language disorders, for whatever reason.

There is another difficulty in drawing conclusions about the cause-and-effect relationship between higher level language disorders and phonological disorders. In random selection designs that have the necessary situation controls, it can be concluded that the independent variable has caused a change in the dependent variable. The causes of HCDs cannot be determined in simple natural group designs. Even if all relevant variables are controlled, there is no way of proving that the phonological disorders were not caused by the higher level language disorder, or that both disorders were not separately caused by another disorder such as dysfunction of the left cerebral hemisphere. Difficulties in reaching conclusions about cause-and-effect relationships are discussed further in Chapter 7.

Natural/matched group designs can also be used to compare two groups of HCDs where the natural groupings are defined by differences in experience. A study might be designed to assess the effects of different methods of training children with congenital sensorineural hearing impairment. A group trained by auditory oral methods and a group trained by total communication methods would be compared in educational achievement. The independent variable would be method of language training and the dependent variable a measure of educational achievement especially adapted for children who are hearing impaired. Variables controlled by matching might include age, gender, years of education, cultural background, amount of hearing impairment, and time of beginning language training.

If all relevant variables could be controlled by matching, differences between groups in educational achievement might be attributed to the method of language training. However, even when the "natural" grouping variable is a difference in experience, it is difficult to control all possibly relevant variables. For example, the two training methods might not be equally available, and the selection of a training method might be influenced by variables such as the child's aptitudes and the attitudes of parents and professionals toward the training methods. Differences between natural groups might be the results of such variables rather than the training methods themselves.

The simple natural/matched group design is often suitable for the purposes of HCD research, but its limitations must be clearly recognized. Matching groups restricts the applicability of the results to groups with the same characteristics, it is difficult to match natural groups on all relevant variables, and a difference between natural groups does not prove that the independent variable has caused the difference. These are very important restrictions for researchers who are trying to fill gaps in knowledge.

REPEATED MEASUREMENT DESIGNS

In the independent group designs described above, the two levels of the independent variable involve two independent groups. In the second type of simple group design, the levels of the independent variable are varied within a single group of subjects. These designs are called *repeated measurement* or *within-group* designs. They are used in HCD research when there are not enough subjects available for two independent groups, when it is difficult to match relevant variables in two independent groups, or when it is more efficient to carry out the experimental procedures with one group. Simple repeated measurement designs may be more appropriate than simple independent group designs for studying the effects of training and for studying changes over time in the dependent variable. The latter studies are called *longitudinal studies.*

The basic rules of the repeated measurement design are simple. The dependent variable is assessed twice in a single group of subjects. The difference between the two assessments demonstrates the effect of the independent variable. Subject variables such as age, gender, and education do not have to be controlled, because the same group is used for both values of the independent variable.

Two examples will illustrate the usefulness of this design for HCD research. If the purpose is to compare the effectiveness of two types of hearing aid, pure tone thresholds can be measured in a group of adults who are hearing impaired with each kind of hearing aid. The relative effectiveness of the hearing aids is determined by the difference in average aided hearing thresholds. The independent variable is hearing aids and the dependent variable is average aided threshold for each aid. There is no need to control subject variables, since the same subjects are tested with both aids, but the conditions of testing the two aids must be exactly the same.

The second example involves the evaluation of training. To determine the effects of vocabulary training on children who are language impaired, a single group of children can be given the vocabulary test before and after training. The difference between pretraining and posttraining vocabulary indicates the effectiveness of vocabulary training. The independent variable is vocabulary training and the dependent variable is vocabulary test score before and after training. There is no need to control subject variables, but the conditions for pre- and posttraining vocabulary tests should be exactly the same.

Repeated measurement designs have several advantages over independent group designs, but they have their own limitations. In both of the previous examples, the repeated measurement of the dependent variable may be affected by the original measurement, which would confound the effect of the independent variable. Repeated measurement effects are called *order effects.* Order effects may take the form of a practice effect that improves performance or a fatigue or boredom effect that impairs performance. When repeated measurement designs are used to assess the effects of training, there is a lack of control for the possibility that improvement might have occurred without training, that is, the lack of a control group with no training.

To control for order effects in the first example above, thresholds should be measured first with one hearing aid for half the subjects and first with the other hearing aid for the other half. This is a control procedure called *counterbalancing* the order of presentation. Counterbalancing cannot be used to control for order effects in training studies, because the pretraining test must always be the first measure.

Even though counterbalancing eliminates confounding by order effects, variability resulting from large order effects or from large differences between subjects could obscure the effect of the independent variable. Such variability can be reduced by extensive practice before the final measurements are made.

To control for the possibility of improvement without training, the independent group and repeated measure designs can be combined, with a trained and an untrained group tested before and after training. This complex design will be discussed in the next chapter.

NUMBER OF SUBJECTS NEEDED FOR SIMPLE GROUP DESIGNS

It would be helpful if the number of subjects needed for a given design could be specified in advance. In general, the more subjects the better, provided that their characteristics meet the requirements of the design. However, when it is difficult to find subjects with the desired characteristics, some guidelines regarding the minimum number of subjects are needed (a more complex method of estimating the number of subjects is described in the section on statistical power analysis in Chapter 16).

The minimum number of subjects for studying treatment effects depends on the expected size of the effect and the expected variability within groups, plus other factors that will be discussed in the chapters on data analysis. The smaller the expected treatment effect and the larger the expected within-group variance, the more subjects are needed. At the time research is being designed it is helpful to have some information about treatment effects and within-group variance to estimate whether it is feasible to carry out the study with available subjects. In the absence of such information, a very rough estimate of the minimum number of subjects for simple group designs is 20. This would require 10 subjects for each of the two groups in independent group designs and 20 subjects for the one group in repeated measurement designs. Smaller numbers of subjects may be appropriate for *pilot studies* that are intended to provide preliminary information in planning further research.

SIMPLE CORRELATION DESIGNS

Another common group design is the correlation design. In its simplest form, two different measures are obtained from each subject in a single group of subjects for the purpose of determining the relationship between the measures. For example, it may be important to determine the relationship between language ability and reading achievement in children who are hearing impaired. A measure of language ability and a measure of reading achievement are obtained for a group of children who are hearing impaired. A statistical analysis indicates the degree of relationship or *correlation* between the two measures. This provides an estimate as to the extent to which good reading is associated with good language ability and poor reading with poor language ability.

Books on research design may not discuss correlation designs as such. Correlations are less definite than differences between experimental conditions. The independent and dependent variables are not usually defined. The degree of relationship estimates the similarity of two variables rather than the difference between two levels of an independent variable.

A major limitation of correlation designs is the difficulty of interpreting the observed relationships. In the above example, the researchers might wish to find out whether reading difficulties of children who are hearing impaired were caused by their difficulties in language acquisition. However, a high correlation between language ability and reading achievement is not sufficient evidence of a cause-and-effect relationship. It is conceivable that reading difficulties cause language difficulties, or that both variables are correlated with a third variable. The degree of relationship also depends on the amount of variability among subjects for the two measures. Where there is restricted variability, the correlation may be smaller.

Because of these limitations, correlation designs are often used to provide supplementary evidence rather than primary evidence regarding a particular HCD research problem.

ADDITIONAL INFORMATION

Simple research designs are discussed in texts on research methods, such as those listed at the end of Chapter 4. In particular, the text by Shaughnessy and Zechmeister (1985) gives a very clear explanation of simple group designs.

• • • • • • • REVIEW QUESTIONS • • • • • • • •

1. List the simple group designs discussed in this chapter.

2. Briefly define each design.

3. Give the main limitations of each type of research design for HCD research.

• • • • • • • • • • EXERCISES • • • • • • • • • • •

(answers are given in Appendix D)

1. In simple group designs, how many independent variables, levels of independent variables, and dependent variables are there?

2. What is the minimum number of subjects for simple group designs?

3. What kind of designs were used in Exercises 1, 2, and 3 in Chapter 4?

4. What would be the most appropriate type of simple group design for the following problems:

Possible personality problems of stutterers;

Evaluation of a new speech aid for laryngectomies;

Comparison of two speech discrimination tests.

5. You wish to determine whether a new hearing aid is better than a standard hearing aid for children who are hearing impaired. Identify the independent variable, the levels of the independent variable, the dependent variable, and relevant subject and situation controls. Design studies of this problem using random assignment, matched group, and repeated measurement designs.

Complex Group Research Designs

In simple group designs there is one independent variable with two levels, and one dependent variable. Such designs can yield useful information about HCDs, as described in the previous chapter. However, the information may be limited. Complex designs can provide more detailed information about HCDs. The complex designs described in this chapter are based on the simple designs described in the previous chapter.

Complex designs are logical extensions of simple designs. There may be more than two levels of the independent variable, and more than one independent variable. There may also be more than one dependent variable. Independent group designs and repeated measure designs may be combined. All of this results in a large number of possible designs to serve the wide variety of purposes of HCD research. Complex group designs make many more research tools available to HCD researchers.

DESIGNS WITH MORE THAN TWO LEVELS OF THE INDEPENDENT VARIABLE

In simple group designs the independent variable has two levels. The two levels used in the examples in the previous chapter were vocabulary training versus no training, boys versus girls, phonological disorders versus normal speech, auditory oral versus total communication methods, hearing aid 1 versus hearing aid 2, and pretraining versus posttraining vocabulary. Researchers often wish to assess more than two levels of the independent variable. For example, more information about age effects is obtained by assessing three or more age levels in independent group designs, and more complete information is obtained about hearing aids by assessing three or more hearing aids in repeated measurement designs.

Independent Group Designs

Increasing the number of levels of the independent variable greatly enhances the amount of information in independent group designs. In a study in which the independent variable is language training and the dependent variable is scores on a language test, the results provide only one piece of information. Children who are language disordered and receive language training will score higher, lower, or the same as children who do not receive training. If the independent variable has three levels—training by Method A, training by Method B, or no training, the results will indicate whether either or both training methods are better than no training, and whether one training method is better than the other. More detailed information about the potential advantages of a training method can be obtained by comparing it with another method, as well as comparing it with no training.

Repeated Measurement Designs

Increasing the number of levels of the independent variable also gives more information in repeated measurement designs. A design that permits researchers to compare more than two hearing aids or more than two levels of background noise would greatly facilitate practical research.

As in the simple repeated measurement design, the effects of order of presentation must be controlled by counterbalancing. The more levels of the independent variable, the more complex the counterbalancing procedure. Each level has to occur at each position in the order an equal number of times. This can be done by complete counterbalancing, using all possible orders. However, the number of possible orders increases sharply with the number of levels of the independent variables. There are 6 possible orders for three levels, 24 for four levels, and 120 for five levels.

An alternative is to use incomplete counterbalancing. The most common technique for incomplete counterbalancing is the *Latin Square*, where each level is presented once at each position in a given order of presentation. The Latin Squares in Table 6–1 could be used with three, four, and five levels of the independent variable (the levels are labeled by letters).

Three subgroups of subjects would be needed to control for order effects with three levels, four with four levels, and five with five levels of the independent variable. As in the simple repeated measurement design, counterbalancing serves as a control for possible confounding of the independent variable by order effects. However, any order effects that did occur, such as practice effects, fatigue, or boredom, could become greater as the number of conditions increased. The increased variability associated with order effects could obscure the effect of the independent variable. Thus, counterbalancing controls for order effects but does not reduce them. It is best to plan a procedure that will minimize practice effects, fatigue, and boredom.

The possibility of more than two repeated measurements also increases the amount of information that can be obtained from training studies and other studies that assess performance over time. For example, assessment of vocabulary training would be more precise if several measures were obtained before, during, and after training. Assessment of the dependent variable several months or years after training has been completed is especially important for practical research. Multiple repeated measurements are also very useful in longitudinal studies, in which a dependent variable such as language ability is repeatedly measured over a number of years in HCD populations such as children who are language impaired and children who are hearing impaired.

TABLE 6–1. Latin Squares Used with Three, Four, and Five Levels of an Independent Variable

ORDER OF PRESENTATION	LEVELS OF THE INDEPENDENT VARIABLE		
	3	4	5
1	A B C	A B C D	A B C D E
2	B C A	D C B A	E D B C A
3	C A B	C A D B	D C A E B
4		B D A C	C A E B D
5			B E D A C

FACTORIAL DESIGNS: MORE THAN ONE INDEPENDENT VARIABLE

For many of the important problems of HCD research, simple research designs do not provide enough information. Even when the complexity of the design is increased by using more than two levels of the independent variable, more detailed information may be needed. Designs that vary two or more independent variables at the same time can provide detailed information suitable to the complexity of the processes and the disorders studied. Such designs are called *factorial designs*.

An important advantage of having more than one independent variable is that the characteristics of the populations can be better controlled. In studying the effect of training method on the language development of children who are hearing impaired, it is important to assess the effects of other independent variables at the same time. For example, both amount of hearing loss and duration of training have important effects on language acquisition. By varying amount of hearing loss and duration of training as additional independent variables, the effects of type of training can be determined more precisely. Language acquisition by the two training methods can be determined as a function of amount of hearing loss and duration of training. The methods may not be equally effective at each level of hearing impairment, and the course of language acquisition may differ for the two methods.

It might appear that HCD researchers can obtain precise information concerning all of the complexities of HCDs by using factorial designs to study all relevant independent variables at the same time. Unfortunately, this is not the case. Factorial designs are very useful, but have their own particular limitations. The more complex the design, the greater the number of experimental conditions or *cells* in the factorial design. A design with two independent variables with two levels each has four cells (2×2), a design with three independent variables with two levels each has eight cells ($2 \times 2 \times 2$), and a design that has four independent variables with five, four, three, and two levels, respectively, would have 120 cells. It is difficult to find enough subjects with the necessary characteristics to fill the cells of complex designs. For example, it would probably not be possible to find large enough subgroups of children who are hearing impaired to fill the cells of a design that varies type of training, amount of hearing impairment, and duration of training.

Interactions

As noted, factorial designs provide more detailed information concerning gaps in knowledge than do simple group designs. Not only can more independent variables be studied, but also, the relationships among the independent variables can be determined. Relationships are indicated by *interactions* between independent variables. In a 2 × 2 factorial design, if one independent variable has the same effect for both levels of the other independent variable, there is no interaction between the independent variables. If the first independent variable has one effect for one level and another effect for the other level of the second independent variable, there is an interaction. This sounds complicated, but a concrete example will illustrate the simplicity of such an interaction.

In a study using a 2 × 2 mixed factorial design, the independent group variable is left frontal lobe versus left temporal lobe brain lesions, the repeated measurement variable is receptive versus expressive language ability, and the dependent variable is scores on a test of receptive and expressive language ability. If both the frontal and the temporal lobe group were most impaired in expressive language, there would be no interaction between location of lesion and type of language impairment. For both groups, expressive language would be more impaired than receptive language. If the frontal lobe group was most impaired in expressive language, but the temporal lobe group was most impaired in receptive language, there would be an interaction between the location of lesion and the type of language impairment. The effect of frontal lobe lesions on language ability would be different from the effect of temporal lobe lesions. The information about interactions could be very useful for planning treatment.

One important advantage of factorial designs, then, is that they provide a way to determine whether the effects of one independent variable are the same for different levels of other independent variables. When the effects vary, they are described as interactions of independent variables. Other examples of interactions are given in this chapter, and also in Chapter 12.

SIMPLE FACTORIAL DESIGNS

The simplest factorial design has two independent variables, each with two levels, and is called a 2 × 2 factorial design. The numbers refer to the number of levels. A 2 × 2 × 2 factorial design has three independent variables, each with two levels, and a 3 × 4 factorial design has two independent variables, one with three levels and the other with four levels.

The two independent variables in the simple 2 × 2 design can both be independent groups, both repeated measures, or one independent group and one repeated measure. Examples of these simple designs will make it much easier to understand the more complex factorial designs.

2 × 2 Independent Group Designs

The 2 × 2 independent group design could be used in HCD research when one independent variable is a natural group difference between HCD and normal subjects and the other is a natural group difference that would provide more detailed information about the HCD. In a study of higher order language skills in children with phonological disorders versus normal children, more detailed information would be obtained with gender as a second independent variable. If the difference in language ability between children with and children without phonological disorders was the same for girls and boys, there would be no interaction between gender and phonological disorders. If the difference in language ability between children with and children without phonological disorders was larger for boys, there would be an interaction. With this particular example, further research might be needed before practical application. To obtain more insight about gender differences, age might be added as a third independent variable in further research.

2 × 2 Repeated Measurement Designs

In studies of the effect of two different treatments on a group with HCD, it might be useful to assess the treatments in different situations. In a comparison of word recognition by adults with conductive hearing loss for two different hearing aids, word recognition could be measured in a quiet situation and a noisy situation. The two independent variables would be hearing aids and noise, each with two levels. The resulting comparison would provide very useful information. There might be no difference between aids in quiet, but one aid might improve word recognition more in noise. It would seem best to choose an aid that works better in noise.

If, however, one aid was found to be better in quiet and the other in noise, patients who needed to hear in quiet would choose one aid and those who needed to hear in noisy conditions would choose the other aid. Those who could afford two aids could use one aid in quiet and the other in noise. The discovery of an interaction between the repeated measurement variables of noise level and hearing aid effectiveness could have very important implications for hearing aid users.

In factorial as well as simple repeated measurement designs, it is necessary to control for order of presentation by counterbalancing. In the above example, at least four subgroups of subjects would be needed. The four orders of presentation could be counterbalanced by a Latin Square procedure, as described previously.

2 × 2 Mixed Designs

The mixed factorial design that uses both independent groups and repeated measurements is very common in HCD research. In the preceding chapter, two different research designs were suggested for studying the effects of vocabulary training on children who are language impaired. The random selection design compared a trained and an untrained group. The repeated measurement design compared vocabulary scores before and after training for one group. More complete information about the effects of training could be obtained by combining the two designs into a 2 × 2 mixed design. In the mixed design, the independent group variable would be training versus no training, and the repeated measurement independent variable would be time of testing. If the groups were similar in vocabulary before training, but the trained group had a much larger vocabulary after training, the interaction between training and time of testing would demonstrate the effectiveness of training.

The mixed factorial design overcomes the limitations of the two simple designs. The use of two independent variables eliminates the possible effects of uncontrolled variables in the simple independent group design and the possible practice, fatigue, or boredom effects in the simple repeated measurement design.

COMPLEX FACTORIAL DESIGNS

The simplest factorial design is the 2 × 2 design with two levels of two independent variables that may be independent groups, repeated measurements, or both. Factorial designs can be made more complex by increasing the number of independent variables, the number of levels of independent variables, or both. There can be three or more independent variables, and three or more levels of each independent variable. Thus, the complexity of the design can be increased to equal the complexity of the process studied. Several examples will illustrate the usefulness of complex factorial designs for HCD research.

If researchers wished to study the effects of linguistic complexity on stuttering, their present knowledge of stuttering might indicate the importance of determining the effects of linguistic complexity separately for subjects of different gender and amounts of education. This could be accomplished by a factorial design that had three independent variables with two levels each, a 2 × 2 × 2 factorial design, as shown in Table 6–2.

The linguistic complexity variable would be a repeated measurement and the other independent variables would be independent groups. The dependent variable would be amount of nonfluency on an oral reading task that included simple and complex passages presented in counterbalanced order.

Complex factorial designs are interpreted in the same manner as simple factorial designs, but there are many more possible outcomes. In the present example, the basic interest is in the effects of the independent variable of linguistic complexity on the dependent variable of nonfluency. Are there more nonfluencies on complex than on simple oral reading passages? This question could be answered by use of a simple repeated measures design with the independent variable being two repeated measurements for one group. The complex factorial design provides more detailed information about different subgroups.

If the total group is less fluent when reading complex passages, does this complexity effect occur to the same extent in subjects of different gender and amounts of education? It might be found that the complexity effect is greater for males than for females, and greater for high school than for university subjects. These would be *simple interactions* between

TABLE 6–2. A 2 × 2 × 2 Factorial Design

INDEPENDENT VARIABLES	LEVELS	
Linguistic complexity	Simple vs. complex	Repeated measurement
Gender	Male vs. female	Independent groups
Education	High school vs. university	Independent groups

the complexity effect and each of the other independent variables. The complex factorial design would provide a great deal more information than the simple design. The finding that the effects of linguistic complexity on stuttering vary as a function of both gender and education could be very useful information for the practitioner.

However, the complex factorial design can yield still more information in the form of *complex interactions*. Such interactions are often considered too difficult to interpret, but there is no difficulty if the logic used to interpret simple interactions is applied to the complex interactions. For the simple interactions, the question was whether the same complexity effect occurred for subjects of different gender and different educational levels. For the more complex interaction, one question is whether the interaction between complexity and educational level is the same for males and females. The complexity effect might occur for both high school and university males, but only for high school females. This interaction between linguistic complexity, gender, and education could also provide useful information for the practitioner. The joint effects of gender and education could dictate different treatment strategies for females but not for males as a function of their education.

Practitioners might believe that even more information should be obtained by increasing the number of levels of independent variables. Three or four levels of linguistic complexity and three or four levels of education might be more informative. Additional independent variables might also provide more useful information. The practitioner might be concerned with linguistic complexity effects before and after treatment. If the effects of different types of treatment were also of interest, still another independent variable would be added.

Very detailed information about a problem can be obtained by using the factorial design strategy of selecting independent variables of interest and varying the number of levels of each independent variable as needed. The limitations of complex factorial designs are the numbers of subjects and experimental conditions required by the design. This depends on the number of cells in the design. The number of cells is calculated by multiplying the number of levels for each independent variable. If there are the three independent variables of linguistic complexity, gender, and education with two levels each, there is a $2 \times 2 \times 2$ factorial design with eight cells. The eight cells would consist of two repeated measurement cells for each of four groups. The four groups are high school males, high school females, university males, and university females.

If the levels of complexity were increased to three and the levels of education to four, the design would become a 3 × 2 × 4 factorial design with three repeated measurement cells for each of eight groups, making a total of 24 cells. If the number of independent variables were increased by varying the type of reading passage with three levels (fiction, nonfiction, and poetry) and the type of treatment with three levels (behavioral, psychoanalytic, and combined), the design would become a 3 × 3 × 2 × 4 × 3 factorial design with nine repeated measure cells for each of 24 groups, for a total of 216 cells.

As the above example indicates, increasing the complexity of the design would soon result in too many experimental conditions and groups, and too many cells in the experimental design. Complex factorial designs can provide very detailed information. Such information may be useful for planning different types of treatment for different types of clients in different communication situations. However, the number and the levels of independent variables must be selected with the greatest of care.

NUMBER OF SUBJECTS NEEDED FOR COMPLEX GROUP DESIGNS

The reasoning used in deciding on the number of subjects needed for complex group designs is the same as that used for simple group designs. The larger the expected treatment effects and the smaller the within-group variance, the fewer subjects are needed. Preliminary information about these values is helpful. In the absence of such information, a very rough estimate of the minimum number of subjects is 5 to 10 subjects per independent group or repeated measurement cell. For example, a minimum of 20 to 40 subjects would be needed for the four cells of a 2 × 2 factorial design and a minimum of 300 to 600 subjects for the 60 cells of a 3 × 4 × 5 factorial design (see also the discussion of statistical power analysis in Chapter 16).

COMPLEX CORRELATION DESIGNS

Simple correlation designs provide information about the relationship between two variables such as language ability and reading achievement in children who are hearing impaired. Like simple independent group or repeated measurement designs, simple correlation designs may not provide enough information. Complex correlation designs provide more information about relationships. These designs are usually considered statistical techniques rather than research designs. They are discussed here as research designs because they provide additional ways of obtaining information about HCDs. The number of subjects required for complex correlations is an important consideration. A very rough estimate of the minimum number is 10 to 20 subjects per variable correlated.

Partial Correlation

If other variables may affect the relationship between two variables, their effects can be controlled by a *partial correlation* design. For example, in studying the relationship between language ability and reading achievement in children who are hearing impaired, it might not be possible to test all children of the same age or to control age by testing different age groups. Both reading and language ability should increase with age. If age effects were not controlled, the correlation between language ability and reading achievement could be confounded by their joint relationship with age. In such a case, the effects of age could be held constant by partial correlation, which would adjust the correlation between language ability and reading achievement to eliminate the effects of their correlation with age.

Multiple Correlation

When there is a need to determine the relationship between one variable and a number of other variables operating jointly, the multiple correlation between the *predictor variables* and the *criterion variable* can be determined. For example, it may be useful to assess the relationship between different levels of language ability (the predictor variables) and reading achievement (the criterion variable). The joint relationship of phonetic, phonological, lexical, syntactic, and semantic ability to reading achievement would be determined by *multiple correlation*.

Multiple Regression

Multiple regression designs go one step further than multiple correlation designs by providing information about the unique relationship between each predictor variable and the criterion variable. This useful information cannot be obtained from separate correlations between the criterion variable and each of the predictor variables. It is necessary to control for the correlations between the different predictor variables by multiple regression. Multiple regression thus combines the functions of partial correlation and multiple correlation.

The multiple regression design would appear to be an ideal method for finding the causes of HCDs. By means of the multiple regression design, the independent correlations between predictor (possible causal) variables and the criterion variable (HCD) could be determined. However, there are limitations to the application of multiple regression designs to HCD research. The demonstration of a relationship between variables is not sufficient to prove that changes in one variable cause changes in the other variable; and the more variables that are correlated, the more subjects are needed. A multiple regression procedure called *path analysis* that does assess causal relationships is described in Chapter 19.

Factor Analysis and Cluster Analysis

Factor analysis is a correlation design that groups variables together on the basis of their interrelationships. In a study of the pattern of language deficit associated with childhood language disorders, a large number of language measures might be obtained in a preliminary study. The number of measures could be reduced by factor analysis without reducing the range of abilities assessed. Factor analysis groups measures that are highly correlated with each other into factors. Then a single measure that best represents each factor can be selected.

After a preliminary factor analysis of the language abilities of normal children, children with language disorders could be compared to children with normal language by using only one measure for each of the factors. The information could be obtained more rapidly, avoiding boredom and fatigue from taking all of the original tests, and the resulting pattern of deficit would be more easy to interpret.

Another form of factor analysis called the *Q-technique of factor analysis* is also useful for HCD research. With the Q-technique, subjects are grouped together on the basis of the similarity in their patterns of test scores. If a battery of language tests is given to a group of children with language disorders, the children will be grouped into "factors" by the Q technique. Children with one pattern of language deficit will be grouped into one factor and children with other patterns will be grouped into other factors. For example, children with particular difficulty on tests of language comprehension might be grouped together in a factor designated as receptive language disorder, and children with particular difficulty on tests of language production might be grouped together into a factor designated as expressive language disorder. Such groupings of children into language disorder subtypes could have important implications for intervention.

Cluster analysis is another method for grouping subjects on the basis of patterns of deficit. The correlational design is the same as the Q-technique of factor analysis, but the mathematical procedures for grouping subjects are different.

COMBINED CORRELATION AND GROUP DESIGNS

For certain purposes it is advantageous to combine correlation and factorial designs. Three types of combined design that have been used in HCD research are *covariance designs*, *multivariate designs*, and *discriminant analysis designs*.

Covariance Designs

In group designs in which it is difficult to control variables that might influence the independent variables, a covariance design can be used to hold the effects of the variable constant. Covariance designs are statistical control procedures that serve a function similar to that of partial correlation. In a study comparing the language abilities of normal children and children with cerebral palsy, it might be difficult to match the groups in age. The covariance design would adjust the language scores of the groups to compensate for the difference in age. This design can be considered an alternative to matched group designs.

Multivariate Designs

All of the simple and complex group designs discussed so far have only one dependent variable. Studies with more than one dependent variable are called multivariate designs. The multivariate design controls for the correlations between dependent variables. If researchers wanted to assess the effects of a treatment method on a variety of behaviors, they could use a multivariate design to compare treated and nontreated groups. The effects of the independent variables can be determined for all dependent variables acting together, and for each dependent variable separately.

Discriminant Analysis Designs

If the object of a study is to obtain a measure that will best differentiate two or more HCD groups from each other or from a normal control group, a number of variables on which the groups differ can be measured. Then a statistical procedure called *discriminant analysis* is performed to calculate a combined *weighted score* that best differentiates the groups. For example, a number of measures of lip, tongue, and jaw movement might be obtained in a large group of babies. Then the measures would be used in a discriminant analysis several years later to compare children who developed phonological disorders with normally speaking children. The proportion that each measure contributed to the total weighted score would be varied until the weighted score that best differentiated the two groups was found. This score could be used to predict which babies were most likely to develop phonological disorders. Like other complex designs, a limitation of this design is that the more variables are measured, the more subjects are needed.

ADDITIONAL INFORMATION

Complex factorial designs are discussed in texts on research methods such as Shaughnessy and Zechmeister (1985) and the other texts listed at the end of Chapter 4.

Correlation designs are discussed in the following text:

Kachigan, S. K. (1991). *Multivariate statistical analysis* (2nd ed.). New York: Radius Press.

and other advanced statistical texts.

Information about combined correlation and group designs is discussed in the following:

Tabachnick, B. G., & Fidell, L. S. (1989). *Using multivariate statistics* (2nd ed.). New York: Harper & Row.

and other advanced statistics texts.

• • • • • • • REVIEW QUESTIONS • • • • • • • •

1. In what ways may complex group designs differ from simple group designs?

2. List the complex group designs discussed in this chapter.

3. What are the minimum number of subjects required for factorial designs and correlation designs?

4. What is an interaction? Give three examples of interactions that might occur in 2 × 2 factorial designs.

5. What are the practical limitations of factorial designs?

6. Briefly state the purpose of each of the complex correlation designs and the combined correlation and group designs.

• • • • • • • • • EXERCISES • • • • • • • • • •

(answers are given in Appendix D)

1. For each of the following problems:

Tell what kind of complex group design (not including complex correlation designs or combined correlation and group designs) is most appropriate (e.g., independent group design with more than two levels of the independent variable, mixed 2 × 2 factorial design).

Give the independent variable(s), levels of each independent variable, dependent variable, and minimum number of subjects.

Indicate counterbalancing requirements.

Finally, for factorial designs, give an example of an interaction that might occur for that particular problem.

a. What is the effect of background noise on the recognition of words presented in isolation and words presented in sentences?

b. What effect does age have on speech perception?

c. What is the effect of voice disorders on the speech intelligibility of males and females?

d. What is the effect of different amounts of background noise on speech perception?

e. Do voice disorders affect vowels more than consonants?

Advantages and Disadvantages of Group Research Designs

The group research designs described in Chapters 5 and 6 provide the researcher with many different ways for obtaining information about HCDs. The levels of an independent variable, the number of independent variables, and the number of dependent variables can be adjusted by the designer to meet the requirements of particular research problems. Factorial designs permit the precise analysis of interactions between independent variables, enabling the researcher to determine the complex relationships that exist among variables affecting HCDs. Further information about relationships can be obtained by the use of correlation designs and designs that combine correlation and factorial designs.

Although standard group research designs are most often used, they do not meet all of the needs of HCD researchers. Information about HCDs can be obtained in other ways by other types of research design. HCD researchers should know when to use standard group designs and when to use other designs. No design is ideal for all problems that concern HCD researchers. Each has its strengths and weaknesses. The advantages and disadvantages of standard group designs are discussed here, and the advantages and disadvantages of other research designs will be discussed in Part II. HCD researchers should be aware of the advantages and disadvantages of all research designs. This knowledge will help them to choose the designs most appropriate for the problems they wish to study and to obtain information of most use to practitioners.

ADVANTAGES OF STANDARD GROUP DESIGNS

Standard group designs were developed to isolate the effects of independent variables, control the effects of other variables, obtain detailed information about interactions between independent variables, demonstrate causal relationships, and generalize findings. When designs are successful in achieving some or all of these purposes, useful information about HCDs can be obtained.

Isolating the Effects of Independent Variables

Group designs systematically vary the levels of independent variables to determine the effects on dependent variables. Independent variables can be groups of subjects, repeated measurements of the same subjects, or both.

Controlling the Effects of Other Variables

Variables other than the independent variables might affect dependent variables and thus confound the effects of the independent variables. Group designs control the effects of other variables by allowing them to vary randomly in random selection designs, by holding them constant in matched group designs, or by systematically varying them in factorial designs.

Obtaining Detailed Information About Interactions

Factorial designs provide information about how the effect of an independent variable on a dependent variable may change as a function of changes in other independent variables. Such designs have proved very useful for studying the complexities of HCDs and for obtaining the type of detailed information needed for practical applications of research findings.

Generalizing Findings

A basic purpose of standard group designs is to generalize information from samples of subjects to the populations from which the subjects were obtained. The conditions necessary for generalization to entire populations are seldom met, because entire populations are seldom available for HCD research. However, limited generalizations are possible in standard group designs. This is an important advantage because generalization is difficult with other designs.

Demonstrating Causal Relationships

When the necessary conditions for causal inferences have been met, group designs can lead to an understanding of the phenomena under study. Three conditions must be met in group designs to permit causal inferences. A change in the independent variable must be accompanied by a change in the dependent variable, the change in the independent variable must precede the change in the dependent variable, and plausible alternative causes must have been eliminated. The third condition is met by controlling relevant variables or allowing them to vary randomly. These conditions are easiest to meet with random selection, random assignment, and matched group designs in which the independent variable is training.

DISADVANTAGES OF STANDARD GROUP DESIGNS

Standard group designs have been borrowed from psychological research, where their function is to arrive at a basic understanding of human behavior. Such designs may not be completely suitable for all HCD research problems. The main disadvantages of standard group designs for HCD research are as follows: difficulty in meeting the requirements of group designs, limitations of information about groups, limitations of quantitative information, inapplicability to practical settings, and difficulty in proving causal relationships. These disadvantages will be discussed separately.

Difficulty in Meeting the Requirements of Group Designs

Under ideal circumstances, groups are randomly sampled from the populations being studied. Situation variables that might affect the independent variables under study are held constant or systematically varied to isolate the effects of the independent variables on the dependent variables.

These ideal conditions can seldom be met in HCD research. Matched groups and natural groups are used instead of randomly selected groups, and relevant variables cannot be completely controlled. Relevant variables can be controlled to some extent by making them independent variables in complex factorial designs. However, such designs often require more groups than are available to HCD researchers.

Compromises in ideal group designs are unavoidable. Matched groups and natural groups are used instead of random groups. Not all relevant variables are completely controlled. Because of the difficulty of obtaining large numbers of subjects with the desired characteristics, groups may be very small, and the number and the levels of independent variables may be restricted. Such restrictions limit the interpretations of results obtained with group designs and decrease the knowledge that can be obtained with these designs. HCD researchers who use group designs must guard against the tendency to interpret their findings as though they had met all the requirements of random group designs.

Limitations of Information About Groups

Even when the ideal requirements of group designs can be met, the information obtained applies only to the group as a whole, not to individuals. To the extent that the trends for each individual are the same as the group average, the information can be of practical use. If there are large differences between individuals, group averages may not adequately represent the characteristics of individuals, and the information may not be useful for practical applications.

Limitations of Quantitative Information

In group designs, the dependent variables are expressed as numerical quantities to permit statements about the probability of the effects of the independent variables. Even when the requirements of group designs have been met and group results adequately represent individual performance, a quantified measure of the dependent variable may not provide enough information. The desired information about HCDs may be difficult to express in numerical form. For example, the operations of the speech mechanism involve complex movements that cannot be easily described in quantitative form, and a single numerical score may not adequately represent complex processes such as syntactic ability.

Inapplicability to Natural Communication Situations

Group designs control the research environment to isolate the effects of independent variables. Information about persons with HCDs obtained under such conditions may not indicate how they will perform in natural situations. The problem of ecological validity is greater for some aspects of HCDs than for others. For disorders such as conductive hearing loss, information obtained in the controlled situations required by group designs may apply to natural settings. However, information obtained under controlled conditions about disorders such as stuttering may not apply to natural settings.

Ecological validity can also be a problem in clinical practice. Changes in HCDs in the controlled clinic setting may not carry over to the natural communication situation. Clinical methods have been developed to facilitate carryover from the clinic to the natural setting. Whenever possible, researchers should attempt to assess carryover from the research situation to natural settings.

Identification of Causes

It is difficult to meet all three conditions for causal inference with the use of group designs for HCD research. The first condition can be met when a change in the independent variable (the causal variable) is associated with a change in the dependent variable.

The second condition is met in designs when an experimental treatment such as vocabulary training is applied, and the dependent variable changes after the treatment has been applied. However, much HCD research involves the measurement of existing variables rather than the measurement of changes resulting from experimental treatments, and causal inferences are not possible.

The third condition is met when all variables that might affect the dependent variable are controlled in order to rule out the possibility that changes in uncontrolled variables caused changes in the dependent variable. This condition can be met only by random group and matched group designs. With natural groups, the possibility that some uncontrolled variables may affect the dependent variable cannot be ruled out.

Designs that do not meet all three conditions can only prove that independent and dependent variables are related, not that changes in independent variables cause changes in dependent variables. Studies that do not meet all three conditions are called *correlational studies* to distinguish them from studies of causal relationships. This is somewhat confusing, because correlation *designs* are different from group designs. However, the use of the term *correlational* does indicate that certain group designs do not permit causal inferences.

CONCLUSIONS

HCD research would be much easier if a few group designs met all needs. However, a variety of group designs and other designs are required. Researchers who use group designs without recognizing their limitations are likely to misinterpret their findings, to the detriment of persons with HCDs. Researchers who reject group designs because of their limitations may fail to use the most appropriate design, also to the detriment of persons with HCDs. Awareness of the advantages and disadvantages of standard group designs provides a basis for evaluating the advantages and disadvantages of the designs discussed in Part II.

ADDITIONAL INFORMATION

The advantages and disadvantages of group designs are discussed in most texts on research methods, such as those listed at the end of Chapter 4.

· · · · · · · REVIEW QUESTIONS · · · · · · ·

1. List and briefly describe the advantages and disadvantages of group designs.

2. Discuss the reasons why researchers should neither completely accept nor completely reject group designs.

Procedures

After research is designed, further decisions must be made about the conditions of the study. These research events are called the *procedure*. They involve exact definitions of the subjects, the situations, the tasks, and the treatment variables. The procedures are just as important as the design. The research contributes useful information only to the extent that the subjects, situations, tasks, and treatments are appropriate for the problem under investigation.

SUBJECTS

Persons who participate in research are now called *participants* in publications of the American Psychological Association, but the term *subjects* is still used in HCD research. The design specifies the kinds of subjects to be studied. Subject selection is an important aspect of the procedure. The subjects should be as representative as possible of those identified by the problem and the purpose. Subject selection is limited by the availability of populations. The variables that dictate subject selection can be independent variables for comparing natural groups, control variables to be held constant within groups, or variables used to match groups. To meet these requirements of the design, subjects are selected according to predetermined *selection criteria*.

Selection Criteria

Selection criteria can include age, gender, education, cultural background, history of treatment, abilities relevant to HCDs, the presence or absence of HCDs, and types of HCDs. Age and gender can be specified without difficulty. Education, cultural background, and history of treatment are easily specified in general terms, but more precise definitions needed for certain studies may be difficult to formulate. Abilities relevant to HCDs may also be difficult to specify. For example, language abilities may have to be defined in terms of measures based on a particular theory of language.

Information concerning age, amount and type of education, history of treatment, and cultural background can be obtained from clinic records, school records, and interviews. Greater care is needed to determine educational achievement and abilities relevant to HCDs. Such information may be obtained from practitioners, teachers, and parents, from standardized tests, or by special assessment procedures devised by the researchers. Judgments of practitioners, teachers, and parents have ecological validity, but may be unreliable. Standardized tests and special assessment procedures can provide more reliable information, but may be relatively crude and lack external validity.

The presence and the type of HCDs can be easily determined for some disorders. The hearing loss involved in conductive and sensorineural losses can usually be assessed by standard audiological tests in children and adults, and by special behavioral and physiological tests in infants. Speech disorders can be assessed by perceptual judgments of clinicians, by standard speech tests, or by acoustical analysis of speech.

Language disorders are not as easily defined, because they involve more central processes for which theoretical explanations are still evolving. Acquired language disorders are defined by evidence of brain dysfunction, clinicians' judgments, standard tests, and special tests. Developmental language disorders are defined by the judgments of teachers and clinicians, standard tests, and special tests.

Obtaining Subjects

After selection criteria have been decided on, it is necessary to determine whether the required numbers and types of subjects can be found. There may not be enough subjects in the most accessible clinics or schools. The researchers may have to obtain subjects from other clinics and schools, sometimes in very distant locations. In such cases it is more difficult to control the conditions for testing and training. Alternatives are to collect data over a longer period of time, waiting until enough subjects become available in accessible locations to meet the requirements of the design, or to select a different design.

Sometimes the desired numbers and types of subjects cannot be obtained. Unless the study is abandoned or postponed, the design has to be modified. The number of independent variables can be reduced, the composition of groups altered, or the number of subjects per group decreased. This restricts the scope of the research and reduces the information obtained about the problem. In some cases, a *preliminary study* or *pilot study* that does not meet all of the requirements of the original design may be carried out.

Researchers must take a great deal of care to select the subjects specified by the design and the problem. This is not easy, but the success of the research depends on how well it is accomplished. Difficulties in meeting the subject requirements of research designs are almost unavoidable. Obtaining useful information with available subjects is one of the most challenging aspects of HCD research.

INDEPENDENT VARIABLES

The research design identifies the independent variables to be investigated. To put the design into operation, these variables must be precisely defined. Variables used as criteria for selecting subjects in some studies may serve as independent variables in others. Such variables would include age, gender, education, cultural background, history of treatment, abilities relevant to HCDs, presence or absence of HCDs, and types of HCDs. Just as in subject selection, some of these variables can be defined in a straightforward manner, and others are less easily defined. Great care must be taken in selecting procedures for defining independent variables of this type, to insure that the levels of the independent variable have as much internal and external validity as possible.

The exact definition of independent variables involves special procedures devised by researchers to a greater extent than the definition of subject selection variables. The procedures may vary considerably as a function of the type of independent variables investigated. Some examples are given below.

Hearing Variables

Hearing variables can be defined by standard audiological tests or by special procedures. These procedures can vary the acoustic and linguistic characteristics of sounds, and the acoustic and linguistic context in which the sounds are presented. Pure tones or complex sounds of different frequencies, intensities, and durations can be presented in quiet or noise. Speech sounds, words, or connected speech can be filtered, compressed or otherwise altered, presented to one or both ears in quiet, or presented with competing noise or speech.

The listening task can require the subject to detect, discriminate, or integrate the sounds that are presented. This can be accomplished by the use of physiological, psychophysical, or psychometric testing procedures. Operant conditioning procedures can be used to test the hearing of infants. Almost all of these tasks are presented in conditions in which background sounds are carefully controlled. Only rarely are hearing variables assessed in natural situations.

Psychoacoustic procedures for assessing detection and discrimination are well established, as are operant conditioning procedures and some physiological procedures such as impedance audiometry. Other physiological procedures, such as evoked response audiometry, are not as well established. Nor are psychometric procedures for assessing central auditory processes involved in integration and perception. The goal of research may be to develop reliable and valid testing procedures so that such procedures can be used in later research on the characteristics of disorders.

In research on hearing disorders, the usefulness of the findings will depend on the validity of the measures of hearing. There is less difficulty in assessing peripheral aspects of hearing, but more adequate theories of central auditory processes are needed to serve as a basis for the development of valid central auditory tests.

Language Variables

Language variables may be defined for language reception, language expression, and communicative interactions. Special procedures may be needed to define a particular level of language such as the phonetic, phonological, lexical, syntactic, semantic, or pragmatic level. Receptive or expressive language variables can be particular language levels in carefully controlled communicative contexts or in more natural communicative settings.

Receptive language tasks can require subjects to discriminate, identify, comprehend, or repeat the linguistic stimuli that are presented at particular language levels, or receptive abilities can be assessed on the basis of interactive responses during communication. Expressive language tasks can require subjects to repeat linguistic stimuli at particular levels, describe pictures, describe past events in their lives, respond to questions, retell stories, or engage in more natural communicative interactions.

A number of standard aphasia tests for acquired language disorders and standard language tests for developmental disorders are available, and new tests are devised on the basis of new language theories. These tests are not as well established as tests of peripheral hearing. Special procedures for assessing language abilities have been devised by linguists and psycholinguists as well as HCD researchers. Neurolinguists devise procedures for relating language and brain functioning.

The procedures used for assessing language are of great importance for interpreting research on language disorders. The problem, the research design, and the exact procedures used to evaluate language interact to determine the kind of information about language disorders that can be contributed by research. The value of the information depends on the ingenuity of researchers in developing special procedures, as well as the research design selected and the nature of the problem.

Speech Variables

Acoustic, linguistic, physiological, or motor characteristics of speech variables may be defined for research on speech disorders. The speech can be speech sounds, syllables, words, sentences, or connected speech in controlled or natural settings.

Speaking tasks can require subjects to repeat words, name pictures, answer questions, tell stories, or engage in more natural communicative activities. Well-established procedures are available for assessing stuttering, voice disorders, and cleft palate. Special procedures have been developed for assessing specific aspects of these disorders, such as movements of the vocal musculature, physiological activity during speech, changes in the vocal cavities, acoustic characteristics of speech, and the effects of communicative demands on speech.

In research on speech disorders there is less problem regarding the validity of procedures, because speech variables can be assessed more directly than hearing and language variables. However, speech involves complex movements and changes in the vocal cavity, as well as complex relationships to language variables, and the speech theories on which research procedures are based continue to evolve.

Treatment Variables

Independent variables in HCD research also include treatment variables. The operations used for treatments and for control conditions involving no treatment or alternative treatments must be specified. These operations include the exact type of treatment procedures, the frequency and duration of treatment, and the criteria for terminating treatment.

Treatments might involve communication aids such as hearing aids and augmentative communication systems or training procedures such as repetition of speech sounds, naming, answering questions, and more natural communicative activities. In addition to comparisons with control groups, the success of treatment can be evaluated by changes in the trained behaviors before and after treatment, *generalization* to nontrained behaviors, *carryover* to natural communication situations, and *maintenance* of treatment effects. Treatments may involve standard clinical methods or special methods developed by researchers.

The evaluation of treatments is a very important type of HCD research. The external validity of treatment methods, that is, the extent to which they improve communication in natural settings, is particularly important.

Other Independent Variables

Alternative modes of communication also serve as independent variables, including visual and tactile speechreading cues, sign language, and augmentative communication systems. Other independent variables relate to the consequences of HCDs. These include procedures for assessing the effects of HCDs on personal adjustment and on educational and vocational achievement. The cultural and subcultural contexts of HCDs are also studied as independent variables.

DEPENDENT VARIABLES

Exact procedures must be specified for defining the dependent variables that indicate the effects of independent variables. Dependent variables indicative of hearing include physiological responses to sounds and detection, discrimination, and identification of sounds by spoken, written, or choice responses. Dependent variables indicative of language include spoken, written, signed, or choice responses to test items, language samples obtained in various ways, and communicative interactions. Dependent variables indicative of speech include speech, movements of the vocal musculature, physiological responses, breathing responses, and the acoustic spectra of speech.

Reliability of Judgments of Dependent Variables

When objective measures of dependent variables are recorded, there are usually no questions regarding the reliability of measurement. When dependent variables are subjective judgments of observers, it may be necessary to demonstrate that different observers make the same judgments. This can be done by having two or more observers record their judgments of an ongoing experimental situation, audiotaped or videotaped responses, acoustic representations of speech, or other forms of spoken response. The degree to which observers agree is called *interobserver reliability* and is usually calculated in terms of the percentage of agreement between observers. In some cases extensive training of judges is necessary to achieve acceptable reliability.

TASKS

The experimental tasks may be standard procedures for determining hearing, language, and speech abilities, or special tasks may be used. The task may be an important determinant of the information needed for the research. If one particular ability is to be assessed without involving other abilities, special care may be needed in selecting or devising tasks. For example, to test vocabulary without requiring spoken definitions from subjects with speech impairment, a multiple choice task might be used in which the subject points to a picture in response to a spoken word.

EQUIPMENT

Some studies require a great deal of equipment and others require very little. This can be an important practical consideration for the procedure. For some research, the main focus may be on designing, obtaining, and assessing equipment. Researchers may have to obtain funds for expensive equipment, appropriate space for housing bulky equipment, and technical assistance for constructing, operating, and maintaining complex equipment, although the increasing availability of computer software has helped a great deal in this respect. Equipment may be used to present tasks, record responses, and analyze findings.

Equipment Used for Task Presentation

Equipment used to present tasks can be clinic equipment such as diagnostic and training devices used for hearing tests, speech and language diagnosis and therapy, and education of children who are hearing impaired. Special purpose equipment designed by researchers may also be used. Visual stimuli may be presented with printed tests, picture cards, slides, videotapes, or computer displays. Auditory stimuli can be presented through earphones or loudspeakers from audiometers, audiotapes, electronic tone generators, speech synthesizers, or computers. Considerable time and expertise may be necessary to prepare and record stimuli. Special calibration procedures may be necessary to ensure that sounds are presented at the desired frequency, intensity, and duration.

Equipment Used for Recording Responses

Spoken responses and communicative interactions can be recorded by audiotape or videotape. Choice responses are recorded by electrical, electronic, or computer devices. Physiological responses are recorded by electrophysiological devices specially designed for hearing, language, and speech responses. Speech movements and breathing are recorded by special electronic and electromechanical devices.

Equipment Used for Data Analysis

Equipment may be needed for various forms of data analysis. Spoken responses may be reproduced as visual representations of acoustic wave forms. The accuracy and speed of choice responses may be directly computed. Certain characteristics of language samples may be automatically analyzed. Numerical averages of physiological responses to repetitive stimuli may be calculated. Statistical analyses of numerical data may be carried out. Such data analyses may greatly improve the sensitivity of data analyses and save researchers a great deal of time.

The Role of Computers

Computers began to play a role in research when laboratory computers became available. They replaced much of the equipment previously used for task presentation, response recording, and data analysis. Relatively inexpensive microcomputers now perform the functions of laboratory computers. Microcomputer software has been developed for synthesizing and presenting stimuli, and for recording, analyzing, and storing data. Of particular interest are computer programs for synthesizing and analyzing speech, analyzing language samples, recognizing speech, and augmenting communication. Such computer applications greatly facilitate HCD research. Further advances in computer software, such as that required for speech recognition, will be put to good use by HCD researchers.

TESTING AND TRAINING CONDITIONS

The situation in which the research is carried out is an important aspect of procedure. Quiet, distraction-free testing and training conditions necessary for some research may be difficult to arrange in schools and clinics. Special testing rooms may be needed for auditory and physiological research.

DATA COLLECTION

Research procedures may involve a specific set of operations carried out by specially trained personnel. Explicit instructions and exact sequences of test operations may be essential to the purposes of research. *Double-blind* procedures may be needed to insure that neither the researchers nor the subjects are aware of which levels of the independent variable are being presented. Special procedures may be needed to minimize the effects of practice, fatigue, and boredom. In general, the researchers or research assistants who carry out the research must be well trained, punctual, and consistent; must understand the processes that are being studied; and must carry out operations exactly as prescribed. Otherwise, the results of the research will not be valid, regardless of the care taken in the design, analysis, and interpretation.

LIMITATIONS IMPOSED BY PROCEDURES

Knowledge obtained by research is limited not only by designs, but also by procedures. The findings must be interpreted with regard to the exact subject, task, situation, and treatment variables that have been defined by decisions about procedures. In almost all HCD research, these decisions involve compromises with respect to ideal procedures. Researchers should be as aware of the limitations on knowledge imposed by procedures as they are of the limitations imposed by designs.

ADDITIONAL INFORMATION

Information about specific procedures is found in published research on the topic in question, where further references regarding the sources of procedures may be given. Computer software used in behavioral research is described in the following texts:

Stoloff, M. L., & Couch, J. V. (Eds.). (1992). *Computer use in psychology: A directory of software* (3rd ed.). Washington, DC: American Psychological Association (see also the journal *Behavior Research Methods, Instruments, and Computers*).

Computer applications of special interest for HCD research are:

McWhinnie, B. (1995). *The CHILDES [Child Language Data Exchange] project* (2nd ed.). Hillsdale, NJ: Erlbaum.

Saris, W. E. (1991). *Computer-assisted interviewing*. Newbury Park, CA: Sage.

Schery, T. K., & O'Connor, L. C. (1995). Computers as a context for language intervention. In M. E. Fey, J. Windsor, & S. F. Warren (Eds.), *Language intervention: Preschool through the elementary years* (pp. 275-314). Baltimore: Brookes.

· · · · · · · · **REVIEW QUESTION** · · · · · · · ·

1. In the research reports in a recent *Journal of Speech and Hearing Research,* find the exact specifications for subjects, independent variables, dependent variables, tasks, equipment, and situations. Note any limitations imposed by these procedures on the knowledge that was obtained.

Data Reduction and Descriptive Statistics

When the procedures have been carried out, the researchers have collected the basic information or *raw data*. The raw data are the measures or observations of the dependent variable, which may be spoken, signed, written, choice, movement, or physiological responses. The first phase of data analysis is usually *data reduction*, the process by which dependent variables are expressed in the numerical form required for analysis. After the data have been expressed in numerical form, the next phase of analysis may be to organize or summarize them to obtain *descriptive statistics* that provide useful information about the characteristics of the data.

DATA REDUCTION

Some types of data reduction are simple and rapid. Others are difficult and time-consuming. Microcomputer programs are available for the reduction of many types of data. Data reduction should be taken into consideration in planning research because researchers may not have the time or facilities necessary for data reduction.

Spoken or Signed Responses: Written Transcriptions

When the raw data are spoken or signed responses, the first step may be to *transcribe* the responses into written form as words, syllables, or phonetic symbols. This can be one of the most time-consuming aspects of the research.

The written transcripts may be classified or coded according to their phonetic, phonological, lexical, syntactic, semantic, pragmatic, or other characteristics. These classification procedures may be simple and rapid, or complex and time-consuming. Simple classifications might involve only the determination of correctness of a repetition response, or the correctness of spoken responses to items on standard hearing, language, or speech tests. More complex classifications might be estimation of vocabulary size, determination of the relative frequency of use of grammatical classes, and assessment of pragmatic skills.

Classifications of spoken responses are often numerical representations of the dependent variable, such as percentage correct phonemes or words, or frequency of use of different grammatical classes, discourse devices, or pragmatic strategies. These numerical quantities can be used for descriptive statistics.

Spoken Responses: Acoustic Representations

Acoustic representations of spoken responses may be recorded as *spectrograms* that show changes in sound spectra during speech. The phonetic and phonological characteristics and the quality of vocalizations may be judged subjectively by direct observation. Microcomputer programs may be used to obtain objective quantitative estimates of vocal characteristics such as hoarseness and acoustic characteristics such as format structure.

Written Responses

Written responses can be classified in the same way as spoken responses with regard to correctness, frequency of usage, and assessment of skills. For certain purposes, the quality of the handwriting may also be assessed.

Choice Responses

Data reduction is simpler for choice responses. The response can be a spoken, written, or button-pushing response to indicate detection, discrimination, or identification of stimuli such as pure tones, speech, pictures, or vibrations. If the responses are spoken or written, they are classified by the listener or reader as correct or incorrect. The speed and accuracy of button-pushing responses can be recorded automatically via microcomputer programs.

Movements

Movements of the speech musculature and other movements can be directly observed, with data reduction through subjective judgments. However, movements are often recorded by sensing devices and displayed in visual form or in numerical form.

Physiological Responses

Physiological responses may be recorded as changes in mechanical or electrical activity that are displayed on screens or printed out to permit researchers to make subjective judgments of dependent variables such as brainstem responses to pure tones. Data reduction may be part of the recording procedure, as is the case for the averaging of brainstem responses to a series of pure tones.

DESCRIPTIVE STATISTICS

Descriptive statistics organize and summarize data, but do not yield probability estimates. They are useful for the interpretation of statistical analyses, or may be the final form of data analysis in studies that do not require statistical analysis. Organization may involve ranking, frequency distributions, and tabular or graphic displays. Summaries involve measures of central tendency and variability.

Ranking

Numerical data can be organized into a more useful form by ranking. Ranked scores are easier to assess than unranked scores, as shown in Table 9–1.

Frequency Distributions

If there is a large amount of ranked data, more useful information may be provided by grouping the ranked data into *frequency distributions*, as

TABLE 9–1. Ranking of Numerical Data

UNRANKED	RANKED
23	4
4	8
13	13
8	23

shown in Table 9–2. Frequency distributions can provide a great deal of information. In Table 9–2, it can easily be seen that the HCD subjects tend to have lower scores clustered in the range of 0 to 19 and the non-HCD subjects have higher scores in the range of 10 to 29. It is also important to be aware of the overlap between groups. Some HCD subjects score as high or higher than non-HCD subjects. When only group means are presented, they may be misinterpreted as indicating that all members of one group are superior to all members of another group.

Frequency distributions also provide important information about the *shape* of the data. The distributions in Table 9–2 are fairly *normal*. The scores cluster around a midpoint and become less frequent on either side. Frequency distributions may also be non-normal or *skewed*. The most common forms of skewed distributions in HCD research occur when the majority of scores cluster at the high or the low end of the frequency distribution. Distributions with a large proportion of near-maximum scores are said to have *ceiling effects* and those with a large proportion of near-minimum scores are said to have *floor effects*, as shown in Table 9–3. It is

TABLE 9–2. Frequency Distributions of Ranked Data

SCORES	FREQUENCY OF SCORES	
	HCD	Non-HCD
0–4	8	0
5–9	11	3
10–14	16	7
15–19	9	13
20–24	2	15
25–29	0	7

essential to be aware of ceiling and floor effects. They decrease the possi-bility of demonstrating the effects of independent variables, because the scores are limited by the ceiling or the floor. Less powerful statistical tests must be used for comparing skewed distributions, and the correlations between variables cannot be adequately assessed when there are skewed distributions.

Central Tendency and Variability

The main trends of numerical data can summarized by measures of *central tendency* and measures of *variability*. Measures of central tendency include *means* or averages, *medians* or middle ranks, and *modes* or most frequent numbers. Measures of variability include the *range* of the ranked measures and the *standard deviation* of the measures. Each of these measures is illustrated in Table 9–4. Because the numbers are dis-tributed in a fairly normal manner, the measures of central tendency are about the same. The average can be rounded off to 6, the middlemost ranked number is 6, and the most frequent or modal number is 6. The two measures of variability assess different aspects of the distribution. The range shows the limits of the distribution by reporting the lowest and the highest number. The standard deviation estimates how much the scores vary from the mean. A standard deviation of 2.83 estimates that 68% of the numbers would fall in a region 2.83 above and 2.83 below the mean. This region includes the numbers 3 to 8. It can be seen that 7 (70%) of the 10 numbers fall in this region, indicating that the standard deviation is an accurate estimate of variability even in small samples when the data are distributed in a fairly normal manner.

TABLE 9–3. Skewed Frequency Distributions

		CEILING EFFECT	FLOOR EFFECT
Minimum	0–19	0	26
	20–39	3	14
	40–59	7	9
	60–79	18	1
Maximum	80–99	22	0

TABLE 9–4. Measures of Central Tendency and Variability

SCORES		
1		Mean (average) = 5.7
3		Median (middlemost ranked number) = 6
3	*Central Tendency:*	Mode (most frequent number) = 6
5		
6		
6		
6	*Variability:*	Range = 1–10
8		Standard Deviation = 2.83
9		
10		

It is always useful to look at frequency distributions, as measures of central tendency and variability do not directly indicate the presence of ceiling and floor effects.

Transformations

Some numerical data are systematically skewed in such a way that measures of central tendency and variability are misleading, and the most powerful statistical tests cannot be used. In such cases, it may be possible to *transform* the scores in such a way that the skewed distribution becomes more normal. For example, if reaction times are the dependent variable, the distribution usually clusters around a minimum reaction time and there is a wide dispersion of long reaction times. The distribution can be made more normal by transforming the reaction times to reciprocals, logarithms, or square roots.

Tables and Graphs

Rankings, frequency distributions, and measures of central tendency and variability can be presented in the form of tables and graphs for easier inspection of trends. For questionnaires and surveys, this form of presentation of raw data and descriptive statistics is often the final stage of data analysis. A great deal of care must be taken in the preparation of tables and graphs to make the information readily available to those who wish to use it. Microcomputer programs can be of great help in this regard.

ADDITIONAL INFORMATION

Data reduction and descriptive statistics take many different forms, depending on the type of research. The most useful information about these different forms may often be found in published research reports. Published reports may also give references for further information regarding specific techniques. General discussions of data reduction and descriptive statistics can be found in books on research methods and statistics. Many microcomputer programs are available for data reduction and descriptive statistics (see the references at the end of Chapter 8).

❖ ❖ ❖ ❖ ❖ ❖ ❖ REVIEW QUESTIONS ❖ ❖ ❖ ❖ ❖ ❖ ❖

1. Why must the requirements for data reduction be considered in research planning?

2. List the kinds of data reduction that may be involved in HCD research.

3. Identify the types of data reduction that were used in the research reports in a recent issue of the *Journal of Speech and Hearing Research*.

4. List the kinds of descriptive statistics that are used in HCD research.

5. What information is given by frequency distributions that is not given by measures of central tendency?

6. Why is it important to be aware of ceiling and floor effects?

7. Find the descriptive statistics in the research reports in a recent issue of the *Journal of Speech and Hearing Research*.

Basic Principles of
Statistical Analysis

$\mathbf{S}$tatistical analyses of research data estimate the probability that the observed effects of varying the independent variable could have occurred by chance. These probability estimates provide a means of deciding how confidently the research findings can be accepted as knowledge regarding HCDs. When relationships between variables are studied, statistical analyses also indicate how closely the variables are related. Information about relationships is more difficult to interpret with regard to new knowledge about HCDs. The basic principles of statistical analysis will be described in this chapter. The statistical analysis of simple group designs will be described in the next chapter. Then the statistical analysis of complex group designs and the statistical analysis of relationships will be described in the following chapters.

Formal coursework in statistics is essential for those who wish to carry out HCD research, and also for those who wish to evaluate research with regard to practical applications. Even when statistics courses have been completed, it is often difficult to apply the techniques that have been learned to HCD research. An overview of the applications of statistical analyses in HCD research is given in this and the following chapters. Further insight into this important but difficult aspect of research can be gained by reading published research and consulting statisticians who are familiar with HCD research problems.

PLANNING STATISTICAL ANALYSES

As far as possible, the statistical analyses should be planned at the time the study is designed. The probability estimates that indicate the degree of confidence in the knowledge resulting from research are valid only when decisions about data analysis are made before the data are gathered. If decisions are made after the data have been examined, researchers may consciously or unconsciously organize or select data that show the desired effects. Such biased data analyses provide false knowledge that could mislead practitioners and persons with HCDs.

There are exceptions to the requirement for preplanning statistical analyses. In many studies it is not possible to predict the shape of the distributions of data. If distributions are badly skewed, alternative forms of statistical analysis may be required; if relationships among variables are complex, additional methods of analysis may be needed to estimate the interrelationships of the variables. Such changes in statistical planning should not introduce bias in the form of reorganization or selection. Researchers must always guard against bias in the same manner that they take special precautions to ensure the reliability of observations and subjective judgments. When statistical analyses are properly planned, the research findings will have maximum practical benefits.

SELECTION OF STATISTICAL TECHNIQUES

Another reason why preplanning is necessary is that the statistical techniques must be appropriate to the design, procedure, and data reduction requirements. As much as possible, decisions about these research events should be made at the same time. If an appropriate statistical technique is not available for a particular set of design, procedure, and data reduction requirements, it may be necessary to modify the study to fit available statistical techniques. Researchers who are not familiar with the full range of statistical techniques will be limited in their ability to plan research that contributes the most useful information. In the absence of such knowledge, statistical techniques can be selected by consulting a statistician, but the global planning that takes all events into consideration at the same time may not be possible.

STATISTICAL POWER

An important consideration in selecting statistical tests is to select the most *powerful* test possible. Powerful tests are those that are most sensitive to the effects of varying the independent variable. In formal mathematical terms, statistical tests are tests of the *null hypothesis* that there is no effect of varying the independent variable. Powerful, sensitive tests are those that most often reject the null hypothesis when there is an effect. If the data are distributed adequately, powerful statistical tests called *parametric tests* can be used. If data are not distributed adequately, it may be necessary to use less powerful tests called *nonparametric tests*. The more familiar researchers are with considerations of statistical power, the more effective their research planning will be. Another important aspect of statistical power is discussed in the section on statistical power analysis in Chapter 16.

STATISTICAL SIGNIFICANCE

The outcome of a statistical test is a statement of the probability that the observed effect of the independent variable could have occurred by chance. In Table 10–1, the independent variable is the occurrence or nonoccurrence of an HCD in independent groups, and the dependent variable is the score on a language test. The HCD mean of 13.4 is lower than the non-HCD mean of 19.0, but the groups are small and the distributions overlap. A statistical test of the observed effect will result in a statement of the probability that the difference between means could have occurred by chance. In planning the statistical analysis, the researchers must decide on the level of chance occurrence that they will accept. In almost all HCD research this level of chance, called the *level of confidence* or the *level of statistical significance* is set at a probability of .05 or .01. The .05 level indicates that only 5 times in 100 would the observed difference between means occur by chance. The .01 level sets the chance level at 1 time in 100.

Because the object of HCD research is to contribute useful knowledge about HCDs, the statistical significance of the findings is crucial. Researchers attempt to design experiments, devise procedures, and select

TABLE 10–1.   Hypothetical Scores on a Language Test

HCD GROUP	NON-HCD GROUP
8	10
9	14
11	18
16	25
23	28

methods of data analysis that will lead to significant differences. The choice of the level of confidence is determined by practical considerations. In the earlier stages of research on a problem, the more liberal .05 or 5% level may be selected to guide further research. In the later stages of research, and particularly when there are large groups of subjects, the more conservative .01 level may be selected so that new knowledge may be accepted with greater confidence. Once the level of confidence has been selected, it cannot be changed. A probability of .053 that "approaches" the .05 level is *not* statistically significant. Similarly, if the .05 level of significance has been chosen, it cannot be said that a difference is significant at a higher level, for example, "significant at the .10 level."

ACCEPTING OR REJECTING THE NULL HYPOTHESIS

When an observed difference between means is found to be statistically significant at the preselected level of confidence, the researchers can reject the null hypothesis, which states that there is no effect of the independent variable. However, when the difference between means is not significant, they cannot *accept* the null hypothesis and conclude that there is no effect of the independent variable. A nonsignificant effect could occur even when there actually is an effect. For example, the measures obtained from a language test may be too crude to demonstrate the effects of language training in a comparison of a trained and nontrained group. Similarly, skewed distributions of scores might reduce the observed effects, resulting in a misleadingly small difference in means.

It is important to be aware of the potential dangers of accepting the null hypothesis. Accepting the null hypothesis is probably the most common error in HCD research. There are practical reasons for wanting to accept the null hypothesis. It is very useful to show that a more rapid training procedure produces the same benefits as a slower procedure, or that HCD groups do not differ from non-HCD groups in certain skills. However, this knowledge cannot be obtained by interpreting nonsignificant differences as proving that no difference exists. More complicated research strategies are needed to demonstrate similarities.

There is an equal danger in accepting the null hypothesis with regard to nonsignificant relationships in correlation designs. Correlational measures of relationships are evaluated according to their statistical significance, but nonsignificant relationships should not be interpreted as a complete lack of relationship. If a nonsignificant correlation is found between hearing loss and amount of noise exposure, it should not be concluded that noise exposure is not dangerous. The measure of noise exposure or the measure of hearing loss may have been too crude to indicate a subtle relationship, correlated variables may have confounded the relationship, or variability may have been limited by ceiling or floor effects.

This seemingly technical point regarding the null hypothesis is of crucial importance for the practical application of knowledge obtained from research. The null hypothesis provides another example of why all research events should be considered in planning research. If the stated purpose of research is to demonstrate no difference between groups or no relationship between variables, the researchers must be aware that this purpose cannot be accomplished by simply obtaining a nonsignificant result on a statistical test.

NUMBER OF SUBJECTS REQUIRED FOR STATISTICAL ANALYSES

As stated in relation to research design, it is important to select enough subjects to meet the requirements for statistical analyses. The minimum requirements vary from a desirable minimum of 10 subjects per cell to an absolute minimum of 5 subjects per cell of the design. A 2×3 design would have 6 cells and require a minimum of 30 to 60 subjects. A $2 \times 3 \times 4$ design would have 24 cells and require a minimum of 120 to 240 subjects.

(Another way of estimating the number of subjects required is discussed in the section on statistical power analysis in Chapter 16.) It is easy to see why the kinds of complex designs that are suitable to the complexity of problems concerning HCDs are difficult to put into operation. It is important to consider the statistical requirements at the time of designing the research. Researchers should make every effort to carry out preliminary research that will indicate which variables should be focused on, and simplify designs to permit acceptable statistical analyses with available subjects.

ADDITIONAL INFORMATION

Most books on research design and statistics discuss the basic principles of statistical analysis. Some texts on elementary statistics are the following:

Harris, M. B. (1995). *Basic statistics for behavioral science research*. Boston: Allyn & Bacon.

McCall, R. B., & Kagan, J. (1994). *Fundamental statistics for behavioral sciences* (6th ed.). Ft. Worth, TX: Harcourt Brace.

Sprinthall, R. C. (1994). *Basic statistical analysis* (4th ed.). Boston: Allyn & Bacon.

✦ ✦ ✦ ✦ ✦ ✦ REVIEW QUESTIONS ✦ ✦ ✦ ✦ ✦ ✦ ✦

1. Give two reasons why it is important to plan statistical analyses at the time of designing the research.

2. Why must statistical power be considered in planning data analyses?

3. What is the null hypothesis?

4. What is statistical significance?

5. Why is the choice of the level of confidence important?

6. Why should researchers not accept the null hypothesis?

7. Why is it important to consider the number of subjects per cell in research planning?

Statistical Analysis of Simple Group Designs

S tatistical analyses of simple group designs estimate the significance of the difference between the two levels of the independent variable. For independent group designs, the significance of the difference between groups is estimated, and for repeated measurement designs, the significance of the differences between two conditions for one group is estimated. The choice of statistical test depends on the type of design and the form of the distribution of responses. If there is a significant difference, the null hypothesis is rejected and it is concluded that there is a probable effect of the independent variable at the preselected level (.05 or .01) of confidence. If there is not a significant difference, the null hypothesis is not rejected, and it is concluded that the effect of the independent variable has not been demonstrated.

INDEPENDENT GROUP DESIGNS

Relatively simple statistical tests are used to analyze the data collected with independent group designs, in which the effect of an independent variable of groups is isolated by controlling relevant variables. These tests can be used with simple random selection, random assignment, matched group, and natural group designs.

A hypothetical study will illustrate the statistical procedures. The independent variable is age of beginning language instruction. A group of 10 children who are hearing impaired and who began language instruction before the age of 2 is compared with a group of 10 children who are hearing impaired who began language instruction after the age of 5. All subjects are 8 years old at the time of testing. The dependent variable is a simple test of language ability—the number of words used to describe a picture. The results for individual children in each group are shown in Table 11–1.

The first thing to note is that there is one score for each subject in each group. The statistical analysis of simple independent group designs is based on one score per subject, no more and no less. All of the information that can be obtained from a simple independent group design is derived from these two sets of scores. The statistical test could not be simply a comparison of group means, because the means do not reflect the variability of the distributions.

Inspection of the data indicates a larger number of words in the picture descriptions of the early instruction group, but a number of overlapping scores for the two groups. A statistical test is needed to determine the probability that the difference between the two distributions of scores could have occurred by chance. The most powerful statistical tests estimate the probability by comparing the difference between means to the variability of scores within each group. This procedure is the most powerful because it makes use of all the data.

It is easy to see how these statistical tests work. If all the children in the early group had received scores of 24 or 25 and all the children in the

TABLE 11–1. Hypothetical Results on a Language Test for Two Independent Groups

	EARLY INSTRUCTION	LATER INSTRUCTION
	34	27
	31	25
	30	23
	28	20
	26	18
	24	17
	22	16
	19	15
	18	13
	16	11
Mean	24.8	18.5

late group had received scores of 18 or 19, the mean difference would be the same but the variability within groups would be much smaller and the probability of a chance difference would be much smaller. If the scores had ranged from 0 to 50 in the early group and from 0 to 40 in the second group, with the same group means, the variability within groups would have been greater and the probability of a chance difference would have been larger. The relationship between differences in central tendency and variability within groups is more easily seen when the distributions are plotted as in Table 11–2.

TABLE 11–2. Distribution of Language Test Scores from Table 11–1

NUMBER OF WORDS	EARLY INSTRUCTION	LATER INSTRUCTION
34	x	
33		
32		
31	x	
30	x	
29		
28	x	
27		x
26	x	
25	Mean	x
24	x	
23		x
22	x	
21		
20		x
19	x	Mean
18	x	x
17		x
16	x	x
15		x
14		
13		x
12		
11		x

The *t*-Test for Independent Measures

A statistical test is necessary for estimating the probability that the difference between distributions could have occurred by chance. The most powerful test for differences between two independent groups is a *parametric test*, the *t-test for independent measures*. The calculations are very simple, and can be done with a pocket calculator or a computer program. The difference between means (24.8 minus 18.5, or 6.3) is divided by a number based on the within-group variance (2.52). The resulting *t* ratio is 2.50 (6.3/2.52), indicating that the measure of the effect of the independent variable was 2.50 times as large as the measure of the variability of the groups. Reference to a table of *t* ratios reveals that the probability of such a difference occurring by chance is less than .05 for two groups of 10 subjects. The difference between groups would be statistically significant if the .05 level of confidence had been selected by researchers, but not if the .01 level had been selected. If the difference between groups had been larger or the variability within groups smaller, the *t* ratio would have been larger and the probability of chance differences smaller.

This simple example provides a good illustration of the importance of planning all aspects of research at the same time. The choice of the level of significance is important. If this were one of a number of studies on the same topic, the .01 level of confidence might have been chosen and the difference between groups would not have been significant. To increase the chances of a significant difference, the variability within groups might have been reduced by more rigorous criteria for selecting subjects, and the difference between means might have been increased by the use of a more sensitive test of language ability. To interpret a significant difference as the effect of the independent variable, a natural groups variable, it must, of course, be assumed that all other relevant variables have been adequately controlled.

This example also illustrates the danger of accepting the null hypothesis. If the .01 level were used, the null hypothesis would not be rejected. It should not be concluded that early language training has no effect on language acquisition, but that the effect was not proven.

ONE-TAILED TESTS

To increase the power of the *t*-test, a *one-tailed test* might have been used. With this procedure, a prediction is made that the two means can differ in only one direction. In the present example it might be predicted that if the groups differed at all in picture naming, the early instruction group would use more words. If this one-tailed prediction were made, the probability of a chance difference for a given t ratio would be reduced by half. In the present example, the probability of chance difference would have been reduced from .05 to .025.

The one-tailed test is a procedure that appeals to researchers who wish to increase statistical power. However, the predicted direction of difference must *always* be specified before the data are collected, and the researchers must be willing to ignore mean differences in the nonpredicted direction. In the early stages of research on a given problem, it is best to sacrifice statistical power and allow for mean differences in both directions. See the sections on Planned Comparisons in the next chapter for a further discussion of this research strategy.

Nonparametric Tests of Simple Independent Group Designs

Parametric statistical tests like the t-test are based on the assumption that the distributions of scores are normal and the variances (standard deviations squared) of the two distributions are equal. However, statisticians have found that with groups of equal size, the distributions can be markedly skewed and the variances quite different without affecting the validity of the test.

Even when liberal criteria for normal distributions and equal variances are used, it may be difficult to meet the criteria in HCD research. HCD groups tend to have more widely scattered scores than non-HCD groups. If the experimental task is too easy for the non-HCD group, their near-perfect scores can result in a ceiling effect, and if the task is too difficult for the HCD group, their low scores can result in a floor effect.

When the distributions of scores do not meet the requirements for parametric tests, *nonparametric tests* can be used. These tests do not assume normal distributions and equal variance. The less strict requirements involve a loss of statistical power. Nonparametric tests are less powerful than parametric tests, because they do not make use of all the information about variability to estimate the probability of differences between groups.

The most powerful nonparametric tests use data that have been transformed into ranks. A nonparametric rank test for two independent groups is the *Mann-Whitney* or *Sum of Ranks Test*. The scores for both groups are ranked together, and the probability of a difference between groups is based on a difference between the sum of the ranks for the two groups. In the previous example, the scores would be ranked as shown in Table 11–3. The sum of ranks reflects both the central tendency and the variability (that is, the overlapping ranks) of the two distributions. When the simple calculations for the Mann-Whitney Test have been carried out, it can be determined that the difference between groups is significant between the .05 and the .02 levels, demonstrating that the Mann-Whitney Test was as powerful as the *t*-test for these particular data.

Nonparametric tests that use frequencies or categories are less powerful than rank tests. For two independent groups, a test based on frequencies is called the *Median Test*. The two groups are compared simply in terms of the number of scores falling above and not above the median for the combined groups. The combined group median in the above example is 21 words. Seven scores in the early group and three scores in the late group fall above the median, and three scores in the early group and seven scores in the late group do not fall above the median, as shown in Table 11–4. The probability that such a difference could have occurred by chance, as determined by a procedure called *Fisher's Exact Method*, is not significant at the .05 level. With exactly the same data, then, the difference between groups becomes nonsignificant when a less powerful test is used.

TABLE 11–3. Language Test Results from Table 11–1 Transformed to Ranks

	EARLY INSTRUCTION		LATE INSTRUCTION	
	Words	Rank	Words	Rank
	34	20	27	16
	31	19	25	14
	30	18	23	12
	28	17	20	10
	26	15	18	7.5
	24	13	17	6
	22	11	16	4.5
	19	9	15	3
	18	7.5	13	2
	16	4.5	11	1
Sum of Ranks		134		76

A nonparametric frequency test that is used much more often than Fisher's Exact Method is the *chi-square test*. This test would have been used for the Median Test in Table 11–4 if the cell frequencies had been higher. Fisher's Exact Method is used only for 2 × 2 frequency tables when cell frequencies are small. If the cell frequencies had been larger, as shown in Table 11–5, the chi-square test would have been used to compare the *observed* cell frequencies with the *expected* cell frequencies. The difference between observed and expected cell frequencies would be significant at the .01 level. The chi-square test can be used when data are in categories, and also when continuous measures have been reduced to categories, as in the example shown in Tables 11–4 and 11–5. It is not restricted to 2 × 2 frequency tables, but can be used for two-dimensional tables with more categories, such as 3 × 4 and 4 × 6.

REPEATED MEASUREMENT DESIGNS

The *t*-Test for Correlated Measures

Statistical tests for simple repeated measurement designs are very similar to the tests for independent groups. The most common parametric test for repeated measurement of two levels of an independent variable

TABLE 11–4. Median Test Scores from Table 11–1

	EARLY	LATE
Above the Median	7	3
Not above the Median	3	7

TABLE 11–5. Median Test with Larger Frequencies, to Be Analyzed by the Chi-Square Test

	EARLY		LATE	
	OBSERVED	(EXPECTED)	OBSERVED	(EXPECTED)
Above the Median	20	(15)	10	(15)
Not above the Median	10	(15)	20	(15)

is the t-*test for correlated measures*. The test is also called the t-*test for paired observations*, and can be used when there are matched pairs of subjects in two independent groups. The statistic is calculated by relating the difference between means to the variability of differences between the paired measures. The greater the number of differences that favor one condition, the larger will be the t ratio, and the greater the probability of a significant difference. In the example shown in Table 11–6, the difference between correlated means would not be statistically significant ($t = 0.83$) because the measure of the variability among difference scores (1.80) is large relative to the difference between means (1.5).

Nonparametric Tests for Simple Repeated Measurement Designs

A nonparametric test for repeated measures that uses ranked data is the *Wilcoxon Signed Rank Test for Paired Observations*. The differences between the repeated measures or paired observations are ranked from smallest to largest without regard to the direction of the difference. Then the ranks for positive and negative differences are summed separately. Once again, the greater the number of differences that favor one condition, the more likely a significant difference. In many cases, this test is almost as powerful as the t-test.

TABLE 11–6. Hypothetical Results of Two Tests for a Single Group

SUBJECT	TEST 1	TEST 2	DIFFERENCE
1	95	90	5
2	86	93	−7
3	90	88	2
4	73	77	−4
5	65	74	−9
6	78	80	−2
7	86	95	−9
8	82	80	2
9	87	87	0
10	72	65	7
Mean	81.4	82.9	

The least powerful test for repeated measurements and paired observations is the *Sign Test*. Only the direction of differences between measures is used; the greater the number of differences that favor one condition, the greater the likelihood of a significant difference.

ADDITIONAL INFORMATION

Additional information about statistical tests used for simple group designs is given in the elementary statistics texts listed at the end of Chapter 10. Simple step-by-step procedures for statistical calculations with a pocket calculator are given in the following:

Bruning, J. L., & Kintz, B. L. (1987). *Computational handbook of statistics* (3rd ed.). Glenview, IL: Scott, Foresman.

Nonparametric tests are comprehensively described in:

Siegel, S., & Castellan, N. J. (1988). *Nonparametric statistics for the behavioral sciences* (2nd ed.). New York: McGraw-Hill.

❖ ❖ ❖ ❖ ❖ ❖ ❖ REVIEW QUESTIONS ❖ ❖ ❖ ❖ ❖ ❖ ❖

1. List the parametric and nonparametric tests used for simple independent group and repeated measurement designs.

2. What is the purpose of these tests?

3. Why can't the difference between groups be assessed solely on the basis of the difference between means?

4. What two measures determine the size of the t ratio?

5. How could each of the values be changed to increase the significance of the t ratio?

6. When can a one-tailed test be used? What is its purpose?

7. When must nonparametric tests be used instead of parametric tests?

8. Why is the Mann-Whitney Test less powerful than the t-test? Why is the Median Test less powerful than the Mann-Whitney Test?

Statistical Analysis of Complex Group Designs

The parametric tests used for complex group designs have the same basic rationale as the *t*-tests used for simple group designs. The probability of chance differences is estimated in terms of the ratio of the difference between means to the variance of within-group or within-condition measures. For complex designs, the parametric test is called *analysis of variance*, usually abbreviated as ANOVA. The statistical ratio used for estimating the significance of the effects of independent variables is the F ratio. The larger the difference between means and the smaller the variance within groups or conditions, the larger the F ratio and the smaller the probability that the difference between groups is attributable to chance.

The requirements for simple designs regarding significance levels, normal distributions, equal variances, and the null hypothesis apply to complex group designs in the same way. The complexity of the statistical analysis varies according to the number of independent variables, the number of levels of each independent variable, and the extent to which there is a mixture of independent groups and repeated measures. ANOVAs are laborious to calculate with a pocket calculator, but microcomputer programs for statistical calculations are readily available.

DESIGNS WITH MORE THAN TWO LEVELS OF ONE INDEPENDENT VARIABLE

Independent Groups

When there are three or more levels of one independent variable, the parametric statistic is *simple analysis of variance*. As was the case for the *t*-test, slightly different calculations are required for independent groups and repeated measures. An example of a simple ANOVA for independent groups is a hypothetical study in which three groups of patients with brain damage are required to name a set of 30 pictures. The independent variable is classification of the patients with brain damage, and has three levels—no aphasia, Broca's aphasia, and Wernicke's aphasia. The dependent variable is number of errors on the picture-naming test. To keep the example as simple as possible, there are only 5 patients in each group (see Table 12–1).

There appears to be a large difference among the means relative to the variance of scores within groups. This can be seen more easily by showing the data in distributed form (see Table 12–2). The distribution of nonaphasic errors is considerably above those of the other two groups, which are closer together. The F ratio is calculated in terms of the difference between groups relative to the variance within groups. The results are shown in Table 12–3.

It is easy to see what contributes to the F ratio. The statistical analysis uses only the 5 error scores for each group. The *total variance* of the 15 scores is 529.40. This is *partitioned* into the *between-group variance* (411.60) between the means of the three groups and the *within-group variance*

TABLE 12–1. Hypothetical Picture-Naming Error Scores for Three Independent Groups

	NONAPHASIC	BROCA'S APHASIA	WERNICKE'S APHASIA
	3	10	14
	5	13	16
	7	15	20
	8	17	23
	11	21	24
Mean errors	6.8	15.2	19.4

TABLE 12–2. Distributions of Picture-Naming Error Scores from Table 12–1

NUMBER OF NAMING ERRORS	NONAPHASIC	BROCA'S	WERNICKE'S
1			
2			
3	x		
4			
5	x		
6			
7	x (M)		
8	x		
9			
10		x	
11	x		
12			
13		x	
14			x
15		x (M)	
16			x
17		x	
18			
19		(M)	
20			x
21		x	
22			
23			x
24			x

(180.80) of the 5 scores within each group. Before the F ratio is calculated, these *variance estimates* are made equivalent by dividing them by the *degrees of freedom* (df), which are 2 (3 − 1) for between-group variance and 12 [(5 − 1) + (5 − 1) + (5 − 1)] for within-group variance. The resulting mean square for between-group variance is divided by the mean square for within-group variance to get the F ratio of 13.66. This F ratio is significant beyond the .001 level for 2 and 12 degrees of freedom.

TABLE 12–3. Simple ANOVA for Independent Groups

SOURCE OF VARIANCE	SUMS OF SQUARES	DEGREES OF FREEDOM (df)	MEAN SQUARES	F
Between groups	411.60	2	205.80	13.66
Within groups	180.80	12	15.07	
Total	592.40	14		

If the within-group variance remained the same, a larger difference between means would give a larger F ratio, and a smaller difference between means would give a smaller F ratio. If the difference between means remained the same, an increase in within-group variance would give a smaller F ratio and a decrease in within-group variance would give a larger F ratio. Thus, it is not difficult to understand how the probability of differences among groups is estimated in a simple ANOVA for independent groups by partitioning the total variance into between-group and within-group variance.

Multiple Comparisons and Planned Comparisons Between Pairs of Means

There remains another important step in the interpretation of significant differences among means for simple ANOVAs. Which of the means significantly differs from each other? The F ratio does not provide this information. It indicates only that there is a significant difference somewhere. Additional statistical tests are needed to determine the significance of differences between pairs of means. A series of t-tests might be carried out, but when a given mean is used in more than one test, the probability of chance differences becomes greater, and the t-test is not appropriate.

When it is of interest to compare all pairs of means, *multiple comparison tests* are used. These tests, which are also called *post hoc comparisons*, *a posteriori comparisons*, or *supplemental computations*, adjust the within-group variance estimates to compensate for the greater probability of chance differences. The most common multiple comparison tests are the Tukey, Newman-Keuls, and Duncan Tests. They are easily calculated because they use mean differences, within-group variance estimates, and degrees of freedom from the ANOVA. Multiple comparisons can be made only when the F ratio is statistically significant. Calculation of the

Newman-Keuls Test for the above data reveals that the nonaphasic patients made significantly fewer errors (.01 level) than the Broca's patients and the Wernicke's patients, but there was no significant difference even at the .05 level between the Broca's and Wernicke's patients.

These findings are confirmed by visual inspection of the distributions of scores of the three groups. The nonaphasic distribution was almost completely separated from the distributions of the two aphasic groups, and the distributions of Broca's and Wernicke's aphasics overlapped a great deal. However, exact probability estimates cannot be made by visual inspection of the data. The simple ANOVA in conjunction with multiple comparison tests provides a powerful statistical technique for estimating the probability of differences among three or more levels of one independent variable. Once again, the interpretation of significant differences as demonstrating the effect of the independent variable—natural groups—depends on how well other relevant variables have been controlled.

An even more powerful technique for estimating the significance of differences among three or more levels of an independent variable can be used when the comparisons among means of greatest interest can be planned in advance. These *planned comparisons* must be based on exact predictions of mean differences made at the time the study is designed, prior to collecting the data. Because all possible pairs of means are not compared, the probability of chance differences does not increase as much for planned comparisons as for multiple comparisons, and a powerful test called the *Dunn Test* can be used to evaluate mean differences. Another great advantage of planned comparisons is that the F ratio does not have to be significant for the mean comparisons to be made.

Because much HCD research involves problems for which there is not enough knowledge for confident predictions to be made, multiple comparisons are used more than planned comparisons. In the present example, it would be of interest to compare all pairs of means by multiple comparison. However, researchers might feel confident enough of their past knowledge to predict that the nonaphasic group would score lowest and one aphasic group would score next lowest. In such a case, planned comparisons could be used to compare only two pairs of means. It would be necessary only to compare the two aphasic groups and to compare the lowest scoring aphasic group with the nonaphasic group; it would not be necessary to compare the highest scoring aphasic group with the nonaphasic group.

Repeated Measurements

Although the calculations are different, the probability estimate for differences among three or more repeated measures is arrived at in essentially the same way as the probability estimate for three independent groups. The F ratio is calculated in terms of the ratio of between-condition and within-condition variance, and additional comparisons between means are calculated in about the same way as for independent groups.

Nonparametric Tests

Less powerful nonparametric tests making use of ranks or medians can be used to determine the significance of differences among three or more levels of one independent variable for both independent groups and repeated measures. These tests are not as useful as parametric tests because additional comparisons of the significance of differences between pairs of means are not possible.

FACTORIAL DESIGNS

The next level of complexity of group designs involves factorial designs with two or more independent variables, each of which may have two or more levels. The parametric statistic used for the analysis of factorial designs is *factorial analysis of variance*.

   In the simple ANOVA there is just one independent variable, and the ANOVA determines whether there is a significant difference between the three or more means. In the factorial ANOVA, the significance of differences between means is determined for two or more independent variables. The most important difference between the simple and the factorial ANOVA is in the *interaction effects*, which do not occur in simple ANOVAs.

Main Effects and Interactions

The tests of significance of differences between the levels of each independent variable are called *main effects*. The interaction effects are essential for the purposes of the research design, because they indicate whether the main effects of independent variables vary at different levels of other independent variables.

If there are two independent variables, two main effects and one interaction are assessed by the factorial ANOVA, as in the following example of a 2 × 3 independent group design:

Main Effects: **Variable 1:** HCD (language disorder versus normal language)

Variable 2: Age (5, 6, 7)

Interaction: HCD × Age

There is an interaction if the difference between language disordered and normal language groups changes for different age groups. This would occur if differences between language disordered and normal language groups were larger at age 5 than at age 7.

If there are three independent variables, there are three main effects and four interactions, as in the following example of a 2 × 3 × 2 independent group design:

Main Effects: **Variable 1:** HCD (2 levels)

Variable 2: Age (3 levels)

Variable 3: Gender (2 levels)

Interactions: HCD × Age

HCD × Gender

Age × Gender

HCD × Age × Gender

Interactions between two variables could occur in the same way as in the previous example. An HCD × Age × Gender interaction could occur if the HCD × Age interaction were different for males and females. This could occur if there were a smaller difference between groups with language disorder and normal language groups at ages 6 and 7 for female subjects, but only at age 7 for male subjects.

If there are four independent variables, there are four main effects, and now there are 11 interactions, as in the following example of a 2 × 3 × 2 × 3 mixed design:

Main Effects: **Variable 1:** HCD

Variable 2: Age

Variable 3: Gender

Variable 4: Language Level (Lexical, Syntactic, Semantic)

Interactions: HCD × Age

HCD × Gender

HCD × Language Level

Age × Gender

Age × Language Level

Gender × Language Level

HCD × Age × Gender

HCD × Age × Language Level

HCD × Gender × Language Level

Age × Gender × Language Level

HCD × Age × Gender × Language Level

Interactions among three variables would occur in the same way as in the previous example. The most complex interaction would occur if younger male subjects were equally impaired at all levels and older male subjects were impaired only at the syntactic and semantic levels, whereas younger female subjects were impaired only at the syntactic and semantic levels and older female subjects only at the semantic level. Such findings could have important implications for diagnosis and intervention. Even aside from the problems of finding the 180 to 360 subjects needed to fill the 36 cells of the design, however, the statistical calculations and the interpretation of the interactions becomes more complex as more independent variables are added.

Error Terms: Within-Group and Within-Condition Variance

F ratios for main effects and interactions in factorial ANOVAs are calculated in the same manner as *F* ratios in simple ANOVAs. The magnitude of the differences between means is related to the magnitude of variance within groups or conditions. The larger the difference between means and the smaller the variance within groups or conditions, the larger the F ratio and the smaller the probability that the mean differences occurred by chance. Within-group and within-condition variances are called *error terms*, because they are the estimates of error against which mean differences are evaluated.

The error term in simple ANOVAs is easily identified, because the total variance is partitioned into only two components, the between- (group or condition) and the within- (group or condition) variance. In factorial ANOVAs, the choice of error term is more complicated because the total variance is divided into many more components, and great care must be taken to select the appropriate error term for each F ratio. The procedures for selecting error terms are described in statistics texts. However, the computer programs used for factorial ANOVAs usually select the appropriate error terms.

AN EXAMPLE OF FACTORIAL ANALYSIS OF VARIANCE

A relatively simple example of factorial ANOVA using fewer than the minimum number of subjects per cell will indicate how main effects and interactions are calculated and interpreted. The example uses a 2 × 3 mixed factorial design with two independent variables, one with two levels and the other with three levels. The subjects are adults with acquired sensorineural hearing loss. The first independent variable is age, with two independent groups of 5 young adults and 5 older adults. The second independent variable is amount of training in speechreading, with repeated measurements of the same subjects after 0, 8, and 16 hours of training the subjects to use speechreading cues. The dependent variable is number of words correctly repeated on alternate forms of a test for repeating spoken words presented face-to-face. The order of presentation of the alternate tests is randomized. The purpose of the study is to determine whether different amounts of auditory training may be needed for persons of different ages.

The percentage of words correctly repeated by individual subjects at each state of training is shown in Table 12–4.

The basic data obtained with this factorial design are three scores for each of the 5 subjects in each of the two groups. From these 15 scores are

TABLE 12–4. Percentage of Words Correctly Repeated

YOUNGER SUBJECTS HOURS OF TRAINING				OLDER SUBJECTS HOURS OF TRAINING			
0	8	16	Mean	0	8	16	Mean
55	76	92	74	50	60	68	59
68	85	96	83	62	71	83	72
42	63	85	63	46	55	68	56
21	87	93	67	20	33	42	32
35	74	82	64	30	40	48	39
Means 44	77	90	70	42	52	62	52
Means of combined groups				43	64	76	

calculated the measures of central tendency and variability used in the factorial ANOVA (more subjects would be needed if this were a real study).

The 2 × 3 ANOVA assesses the statistical significance of the two main effects for age and amount of training, plus the interaction between age and amount of training. The main effect for the between-group variable of age is shown by the mean for each group, 70% correct for the younger subjects and only 52% correct for the older subjects. The main effect for the repeated measurement of hours of training is the mean of the combined groups, 43% for 0 hours, 64% for 8 hours, and 76% for 16 hours, a steady improvement with training.

It is important to note that the main effect for one independent variable is obtained by *pooling* the levels of the other independent variable. The main effect for age is obtained by pooling the results of the three amounts of training, and the main effect for training is obtained by pooling the two ages.

The researchers' interest is not confined to main effects. They wish to determine not only if there is a significant difference in performance with age (main effect for age) and an improvement with practice (main effect for hours of training), but also whether both groups improve at the same rate. This important information is indicated by the interaction of age and hours of training. The interaction can be seen by comparing the change in the means of the two groups at each stage of training, as shown in Figure 12–1.

There is an apparent interaction. Both groups begin training at about the same level of accuracy, but the younger subjects improve much more than

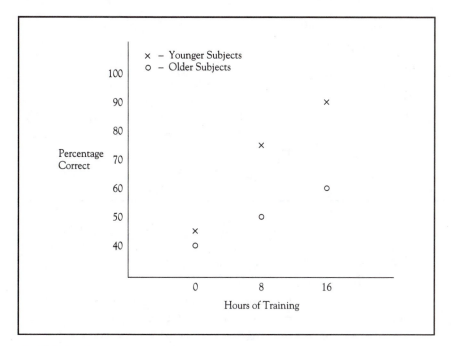

FIGURE 12–1.   Interaction between age and amount of training.

the older ones. The study appears to have resulted in interesting and important findings. However, the amount of within-group variance associated with each mean is not shown. It is necessary to analyze the data statistically to demonstrate that the observed trends have not occurred by chance.

Results of the ANOVA

The results of the ANOVA for the 2 × 3 mixed factorial design are shown in Table 12–5. Table 12–5 is organized differently from the simple ANOVA table (Table 12–3). The sums of squares are omitted, and the level of significance (*p*) of the *F* ratios is given. The main effect of age is not significant at the .05 level (when the symbol points to the right [p >] it means "probability greater than," and when it points to the left [p <] it means "probability less than"). Although there was a large difference between the group means, the distributions of the scores of the small groups overlapped and the main effect for groups was not significant. The main effect for hours of training was significant beyond

TABLE 12–5. Results of the ANOVA for the 2 × 3 Mixed
Factorial Design

SOURCE OF VARIANCE	df	MEAN SQUARES	F	p
Age (A)	1	2576	5.18	$(p > .05)$
Hours of training (T)	2	2776	44.80	$(p < .01)$
Age × Training interaction (AT)	2	480	7.75	$(p < .01)$
Error term for A	8	498		
Error term for T and AT	16	62		

the .01 level. Performance of the two groups averaged together improved with training. The interaction of groups and training was significant beyond the .01 level, apparently because the younger subjects improved more with training.

The Source of Variance column in Table 12–5 has more entries than the corresponding column in the simple ANOVA table (Table 12–3), where only the between-group and within-group variances contribute to the total variance. In the factorial ANOVA, the F ratio is still calculated in terms of the ratio of between-(group or condition) and within- (group or condition) variance. For age, there is a large mean square because a large proportion of the total variance is attributable to the large difference between the group means (70 and 52), but there is also a relatively large variance between subjects within groups (Error Term for A). The error term is based on the variance between subjects with the variance between age groups removed. Thus, the F ratio for age is based on the same type of ratio of between-group and within-group variance as the t-test.

The F ratio for the main effect of training is calculated according to the same rationale. There is a large mean square for training because much of the total variance is attributable to the large mean differences between hours of training for combined groups (43, 64, and 76). The F ratio is calculated by comparing the variance among the mean hours of training for the combined groups to the relatively small variance among training conditions for each subject with the variance between training conditions removed (Error term for T and AT). This variance was small because each subject improved from 0 to 8 and from 8 to 16 hours.

The F ratio for the interaction is most easily understood in terms of *residual variance*. There is a total variance among the means for each training period for each group. The variance among these six means can be partitioned into the variance of the two main effects and the interaction. The two main effects were quite large and took up a large proportion of the total variance, as shown by their large mean squares. The variance among the six means not attributable to the differences between age groups and among training conditions is the residual variance attributable to the interaction of groups and training conditions.

The residual variance can be seen by examining the graphic representation of the interaction in Figure 12–1. If the difference between groups had been exactly the same for all three training conditions, there would have been no residual variance and no interaction. All of the variance among the six means would have been attributable to the two main effects. However, there was a very small difference between groups at 0 hours training and a very large difference at 16 hours training. This residual variance resulted in a significant interaction between the two independent variables of age and amount of training.

It is important to understand the concept of partitioning variance into components and the concept of residual variance because they apply to the calculation of all interactions in factorial designs. In factorial designs with more than two independent variables, there are many more interactions, but the partitioning of variance among main effects and interactions occurs in the same way.

Interpretation of Main Effect and Interaction

If an interaction is significant, the main effects need not be interpreted, because they are explained by the interaction. This can be seen in the present study. The main effect of groups was not of primary interest because it involved a comparison of group means pooled across hours of training, and the main effect of hours of training was not of primary interest because it compared means pooled across groups. If the interaction had not been significant, however, significant main effects would provide useful information about the effects of age and training.

Multiple Comparisons and Planned Comparisons

If the interaction had not been significant, additional computations would have been needed to interpret the significant main effect of training, because the significant F ratio does not indicate which of the differences among the three means were significant. A multiple comparison test of the type described for the simple ANOVA is needed. A Tukey test revealed that the scores of the pooled groups increased significantly (.01 level) from 0 to 8 hours training and from 8 to 16 hours training.

In a study like the present one, the significant interaction can be interpreted by inspecting the pattern of mean differences. It can be concluded that the younger subjects' performance was only slightly better than that of the older subjects before training began, but showed greater improvement with training. If the trends had been less clear, however, further statistical analysis would have been needed. A multiple comparison test would make all possible comparisons among the six means, with the error term adjusted to compensate for the increased probability of chance differences.

A Tukey test was used as the test for multiple comparisons. There was a significant increase (.01 level) in scores for the young group from 0 to 8 hours training, but the increase from 8 to 16 hours was not significant. For the older group, only the increase from 0 to 16 hours was significant (.01 level). The differences between the two groups were significant (.01 level) at both 8 and 16 hours, but not at 0 hours. The remaining comparisons were between groups at different hours of training. The only comparisons of interest revealed that the mean for the older group was significantly higher (.05 level) at 16 hours but not at 8 hours than the mean for the young group at 0 hours training.

The multiple comparisons provide a great deal of information. Both groups significantly improved during training, but at different rates. At the beginning they were not significantly different, but the young group obtained significantly larger scores than the older group after training had begun. The older group's scores did not significantly exceed the younger group's pretraining scores until they had had 16 hours of training. The extent to which this information can be used depends on the purpose of the study. If the researchers only wish to assess the progress of each group separately or to compare groups at each stage of training, more powerful planned comparisons could be used. If in addition to these comparisons, they also wanted to compare one group at one stage of training with the other group at another stage of training, multiple comparisons would be necessary.

The choice of the method for additional statistical comparisons of interactions illustrates the close relationship between the exact purpose of the study and the data analysis. If on the basis of previous research, the researchers had decided that the purpose of the research was to assess the progress of each group and to compare groups at each stage, only these planned comparisons of the means would be made. The increased statistical power would permit a more sensitive test of the training effects for each group.

When the present data were analyzed by planned comparisons of the training effects for each group, the increased statistical power revealed a significant increase in the scores of the young group from 0 to 8 hours (.01 level) but not from 8 to 16 hours (p > .05). This result had also been found with the multiple comparisons. However, the planned comparisons revealed a significant increase (.01 level) in the older group's scores from 0 to 8 hours and from 8 to 16 hours. Inspection of the individual scores indicates that the lack of significant increase from 8 to 16 hours for the young group was the result of a ceiling effect. After 16 hours of training, the younger subjects approached perfect scores on the word repetition test. This finding, which was not revealed as clearly by the multiple comparison test, would be important for planning further research. If more training were to be given, more difficult tests would be needed for valid comparisons of the proficiency of younger and older subjects.

Planned comparisons are most useful when researchers have enough prior knowledge to decide on very specific purposes, and multiple comparisons are most useful when the researchers must rely more on guesswork concerning the outcome of the research. For the present example, the choice of the method of additional comparisons would depend on the amount and type of previous knowledge of researchers and practitioners about auditory training.

Relationship Between Factorial ANOVA and Other Research Events

This relatively simple factorial ANOVA is an excellent example of how all research events are interrelated. The results of the ANOVA could not be fully interpreted without reference to the purpose of the experiment. The factorial design could have served many different purposes. At least five separate studies were nested in the 2 × 3 design. The older and younger subjects could be compared for three different amounts of training, the equivalent of three separate independent group designs. The three training conditions could be assessed for each group, the equivalent of two single-factor repeated measure designs. Putting all of these separate designs together in one factorial design permitted a detailed comparison of the interactive effects of the two independent variables.

A MORE COMPLEX FACTORIAL DESIGN

An example of a factorial design with three independent variables will indicate how ANOVAs involving more than one interaction are analyzed and interpreted. To keep the example as simple and clear as possible, a somewhat artificial hypothetical study will be used, with fewer than the minimum number of subjects per cell.

Assume that the researchers want to find out whether developmental language disorders are associated with (not "caused by") deficient functioning of the left cerebral hemisphere. The left hemisphere seems to subserve language processes in most normal right-handed individuals (note cautious terminology). Tests called *dichotic listening tests* show that when two linguistic stimuli are presented simultaneously to the two ears, recognition accuracy tends to be better for the right ear, which has its strongest connections to the left cerebral hemisphere; and when certain nonlinguistic stimuli such as environmental sounds are presented simultaneously to the two ears, recognition accuracy tends to be better for the left ear, which has its strongest connections to the right cerebral hemisphere.

The researchers decide to attack the problem of whether the "language" hemisphere of right-handed children with language disorder is functioning normally by giving them a test in which pairs of one-syllable words are presented simultaneously to the two ears. If they do not perform better with the right ear, it may be that their left hemisphere is not performing properly. This study could be done with a simple repeated measurement design with two levels of one independent variable (ears). However, proving no difference would require accepting the null hypothesis. This would be inadvisable. Among other reasons, there might be no difference because the test was not sensitive enough to show the effect.

To control for test sensitivity and provide a better means of interpreting a lack of difference between ears, the researchers could also test a control group of right-handed nondisordered children. If the nondisordered children showed the expected right-ear superiority and the children with language disorder did not, it would suggest a difference in the functioning of the left hemisphere of the children with language disorder. This design would be a 2 × 2 factorial design with two independent variables, one involving two independent groups (children with and without language disorder) and the other involving repeated measurement of the two ears. The researchers would predict a significant interaction of ears and groups, where the normal children showed right-ear superiority but the children with language disorder did not.

To rule out the possibility that the deficiency of the children with language disorder involved both cerebral hemispheres, the researchers could give another test for the recognition of pairs of environmental sounds presented to the two ears. The children with language disorder should have the same left-ear superiority as the normal children on this task, indicating normal functioning of the "nonlanguage" hemisphere. If only the nonverbal test were given to the two groups and both had a left-ear advantage, a 2 × 2 mixed factorial ANOVA would show a main effect for ears but no interaction between ears and groups.

A design in which both the verbal and the nonverbal tests are given to both groups combines two 2 × 2 factorial designs. In the design involving the verbal test, the researchers expect a significant interaction, but in the design involving the nonverbal test, they do not expect a significant interaction. Putting the two designs together makes a 2 × 2 × 2 mixed factorial design. If, as expected, there were a Groups × Ears interaction for the verbal task but not for the nonverbal task, there could be a significant interaction of Groups × Ears × Tasks. The purpose of this example is to show that such complex interactions, which may occur more often than simple interactions in HCDs, can be interpreted in as simple and logical a manner as simple interactions.

The minimum number of subjects for the eight cells of the 2 × 2 × 2 design would be 40 to 80. In this hypothetical study, only 8 subjects were used to simplify the interpretation of the raw data. Significant effects occurred because the artificial data were created to exhibit very consistent trends. The two groups of 4 right-handed subjects were matched on relevant variables. Each subject was given both tests, with the order of tests counterbalanced.

The percentage of correct responses of individual subjects for each ear on each task is shown in Table 12–6. Table 12–6 contains all the information needed for calculation of the ANOVA and the descriptive statistics used for the interpretation of the ANOVA. The scores of individual subjects are given in four columns and include one score for each ear on each test. These 32 scores are the raw data obtained with the 2 × 2 × 2 factorial design. The factorial ANOVA partitions the variance among these 32 scores to obtain the between-means variance estimates and the error terms for the main effects and interactions.

TABLE 12–6. Hypothetical Results for a Factorial Design with Three Independent Variables

	WORD TEST		SOUND TEST	
	RIGHT EAR	LEFT EAR	RIGHT EAR	LEFT EAR
Normal	73	45	44	85
language	84	37	36	77
	86	36	34	84
	75	45	43	75
Language	37	46	45	75
disorder	46	34	33	84
	35	36	43	72
	46	44	45	85

The trends can be seen by looking at the individual test scores. The normal subjects scored consistently higher on the right ear on the words task and on the left ear on the sounds task. The subjects with language disorder showed the same trend as the normal subjects on the sounds task, but no consistent ear difference on the words task. The comparisons between groups can be summarized by noting that they differed on only one of four repeated measures, the right-ear score on the words task. This one difference will lead to a significant Groups × Ears × Tasks interaction. The interaction could be interpreted as suggesting that children with language disorder have a specific deficit in left-hemisphere functioning.

The means for the various conditions are the descriptive statistics needed to interpret the main effects and interactions. The means that indicate the main effects and interactions are shown in Table 12–7.

The means are similar because the data were created to show the complex interactions in as clear a manner as possible. The trends of greatest interest are shown by the Group × Ear × Task means. The normal language group has a right-ear advantage for words and a left-ear advantage for sounds. The language disorder group has a left-ear advantage for sounds but no difference between ears for words.

Results of the ANOVA

For simplicity, the ANOVA table has been condensed in Table 12–8. All of the main effects and interactions are significant beyond the .01

TABLE 12–7. Means Showing Main Effects and Interactions for Data in Table 12–6

Combined mean for all subjects (all scores pooled)				55
Group means (pooled ears and tasks)		Normal language		60
		Language disorder		50
Ear means (pooled groups and tasks)		Right ear		50
		Left ear		60
Task means (pooled groups and ears)		Dichotic words		50
		Dichotic sounds		60
Group × Ear means (pooled tasks)		Normal:	Right ear	59
			Left ear	61
		Disorder:	Right ear	41
			Left ear	60
Group × Task means (pooled ears)		Normal:	Words	60
			Sounds	60
		Disorder:	Words	41
			Sounds	60
Ear × Task means (pooled groups)		Words:	Right ear	60
			Left ear	40
		Sounds:	Right ear	40
			Left ear	80
Group × Ear × Task means	Normal:	Words:	Right ear	80
			Left ear	41
		Sounds:	Right ear	39
			Left Ear	80
	Disorder:	Words:	Right ear	41
			Left ear	40
		Sounds:	Right ear	42
			Left ear	79

level. When a higher order interaction is significant, it is unnecessary to interpret the main effects and lower order interactions. In the present study, all of the information concerning the effects of the independent variables is contained in the means for the GET interaction. Because each independent variable had only two levels, no additional comparisons are needed. Both groups had a left-ear advantage on the sounds test, but only the normal language group had a right-ear advantage on

TABLE 12–8. Summary of Analysis of Variance

SOURCE	df	F
Groups (G)	1	25.20*
Ears (E)	1	25.03*
Tasks (T)	1	75.10*
Groups × Ears	1	19.56*
Groups × Tasks	1	81.00*
Ears × Tasks	1	145.90*
Groups × Ears × Tasks	1	13.97*

*$p < .01$.

the words test. This finding confirms the prediction that subjects with language disorder would not show evidence of left-hemisphere dominance for language.

Although the significant GET interaction contains all of the necessary information about the study, it is useful to interpret all main effects and interactions with reference to studies in which the highest order interaction is not significant. Because each of the main effects had only two levels of the independent variable, the significant effects can be directly interpreted without multiple comparison tests. The significant main effects for groups (means of 60 for the normal language group and 50 for the language disorder group), tasks (50 for the words task and 60 for the sounds task), and ears (50 for the right ear and 60 for the left ear), were all attributable to the lower right-ear scores of the language disordered group on the words task.

The significant lower order interactions were also attributable to the lower right-ear word score for the language disorder group (Table 12–9). In the first two interactions, there would be no interaction if the right-ear mean for the language disorder group were not lower. In the third interaction, there would be an even larger interaction between ears and tasks if the right-ear word score of the language disorder group had been the same as that for the normal language group. The right-ear word mean would have been 80, and the Ear × Task interaction would have involved a complete reversal.

The interpretations of main effects and interactions are rendered unnecessary by the significant higher order interaction (Table 12–10). The normal language group shows the expected reversal of right- and

TABLE 12–9. Lower Order Interactions

GROUP × EAR INTERACTION	RIGHT EAR	LEFT EAR
Normal language	59	61
Language disorder	41	60
GROUP × TASK INTERACTION	**WORDS**	**SOUNDS**
Normal language	60	60
Language disorder	41	60
EAR × TASK INTERACTION	**RIGHT EAR**	**LEFT EAR**
Words	60	40
Sounds	40	80

left-ear scores for the two tasks. If this had been a study of normal subjects only, there would have been a highly significant interaction between tasks and ears. The language disorder group did not have this reversal since there were no ear differences on the words task. If this had been a study of subjects with language disorder only, they might still have had a significant interaction between ears and tasks, but it would have been smaller than that for normal group. The interaction of Group × Task × Ear occurred because of a predicted but relatively subtle difference between the Task × Ear interactions of the two groups.

Interpretation

Like the simpler 2 × 3 factorial design, the 2 × 2 × 2 design is very thorough. It partitions the variance of the 32 numbers arising from the four

TABLE 12–10. Higher Order Interaction Between Groups, Ears, and Tasks

	NORMAL LANGUAGE			LANGUAGE DISORDER	
	RIGHT EAR	LEFT EAR		RIGHT EAR	LEFT EAR
Words	80	41	Words	41	40
Sounds	39	80	Sounds	42	79

scores for the 8 subjects into main effects and interactions and isolates the effect of interest in the higher order interaction. As before, the interpretation of the analysis depends on the adequacy of the design and procedure, as well as the exact purposes of the research.

The data of this artificial study were carefully selected to produce trends that could be easily interpreted. For an actual study, 20 to 40 subjects per group would be needed to fulfill the minimum requirement of 5 to 10 subjects per cell. Ear differences would not be uniform, as dichotic tests are open to many sources of difficulty. Assuming that all of the potential design and procedural problems had been solved, the study would have indicated that certain verbal stimuli were not processed efficiently by the left cerebral hemisphere of children with language disorder. Further research would be needed to bring out the implications for intervention.

NONPARAMETRIC TESTS FOR FACTORIAL DESIGNS

There are no nonparametric tests for factorial designs that permit the assessment of interactions.

OTHER ANALYSES OF VARIANCE

Two additional procedures for analyzing the results of complex designs, analysis of covariance (ANCOVA) and multivariate analysis of variance (MANOVA), are discussed in the next chapter. They both involve correlational analysis as well as analysis of variance.

ADDITIONAL INFORMATION

Statistical analyses of complex group designs are discussed in advanced statistics texts such as the following:

Bogartz, R. S. (1994). *An introduction to the analysis of variance.* Westport, CT: Praeger.
Edwards, L. K. (1993). *Applied analysis of variance in behavioral sciences.* New York: Marcel Decker.

✦ ✦ ✦ ✦ ✦ ✦ ✦ REVIEW QUESTIONS ✦ ✦ ✦ ✦ ✦ ✦ ✦

1. Why are additional statistical tests needed for simple analysis of variance?

2. How is the total variance partitioned in simple ANOVA?

3. What determines the size of the F ratio in simple ANOVA?

4. What is the difference between multiple comparisons and planned comparisons in simple ANOVA?

5. What determines whether multiple comparisons or planned comparisons will be used to interpret simple ANOVA?

6. What is meant by the term *residual variance* in factorial ANOVA?

✦ ✦ ✦ ✦ ✦ ✦ ✦ ✦ ✦ EXERCISES ✦ ✦ ✦ ✦ ✦ ✦ ✦ ✦ ✦
(answers are given in Appendix D)

1. List the main effects and interactions for each of the following designs:

   a. Effectiveness of two hearing aids for speech discrimination in quiet and noise.

   b. Effects of age, gender, and speaking task (picture description versus story retelling) on articulation errors of children without HCDs.

   c. Effects of age, education, amount of training, and amount of hearing impairment on speechreading in adults with sensorineural loss.

2. Give an example of a significant interaction that might occur for the highest order interaction in each of the three designs listed in Exercise 1.

Statistical Analysis of Relationships

Τhis chapter is concerned with methods for analyzing relationships in correlation designs and in combined correlation and group designs. These methods involve complex calculations, but microcomputer statistical programs are available for all of the methods. Relationships are evaluated in estimating the degree of *covariance* or *nonindependence* of variables in correlation designs. When two or more variables are assessed for the same group of subjects, the variables covary or are nonindependent to the extent that changes in one variable tend to be accompanied by changes in the other variable. The *correlation* between variables is usually expressed in terms of a *correlation coefficient* that varies between 1.00 and −1.00. A high correlation or strong relationship can be either positive or negative. A positive correlation, for example, between height and weight, would tend to approach 1.00, and a negative correlation, for example, between age and reaction time in children, would tend to approach −1.00. If there is no relationship, that is, if the two variables are independent, the correlation would tend to approach .00.

Correlations can serve as a basis for predictions. The higher the correlation between the predicting and the predicted variable, the better the prediction. The term *regression* is used to describe the estimation or prediction of one variable by another variable. This aspect of the analysis of relationships can have practical importance for HCDs, if some aspect of an HCD can be predicted by the measurement of a particular variable or set of variables.

As noted, the limitation of information about relationships is that covariation, correlation, and regression cannot be used as proof that a change in one variable has caused a change in another variable. Covariation is only one of the three conditions required for the demonstration of causality. The other two conditions are that the change in one variable preceded the change in the other variable, and that plausible alternative causal variables have been ruled out. The latter condition is difficult to achieve in research involving the statistical analysis of relationships. If a strong relationship is found between two variables, it is always possible that both variables are correlated with a third variable. It is very difficult to reach definite conclusions on the basis of correlational analysis alone. Therefore, correlational analyses are often used in conjunction with other types of data analyses.

Statistical analyses of relationships range from simple and easily understood correlations between two variables to complex multivariate correlation analyses. Some of the most representative forms of correlation analysis will be briefly described here. All correlation analyses are based on the reasoning used to interpret simple correlations and partial correlations. It is important, therefore, to thoroughly understand simple correlations and partial correlations.

SIMPLE CORRELATIONS OF TWO VARIABLES

A simple correlation estimates the degree of relationship, that is, the amount of covariance, of two variables. A hypothetical study in which scores were obtained on two different speech discrimination tests for 10 subjects can be used as an example. The pairs of scores are repeated measurements of the same subjects, expressed as percentage correct, as shown in Table 13–1. In this set of data, subjects tend to have about the same score on both tests. This can be seen in a two-dimensional *scatter plot*, where the Test 1 score of each subject is plotted on the vertical scale and the Test 2 score is plotted on the horizontal scale (see Figure 13–1). The scatter plot shows that scores on one test *tend to be* accompanied by high scores on the other. Scores on the two tests are positively correlated. The strength of the tendency for a positive relationship is expressed by the correlation coefficient.

The most powerful test for simple correlations is a parametric test called the *Pearson product moment correlation*. The correlation coefficient, which is denoted by r, is based on the degree of covariance of the pairs of scores relative to the variance within each set of scores. The greater the

TABLE 13–1. Hypothetical Results for Two Speech Discrimination Tests

SUBJECT	TEST 1	TEST 2
1	95	90
2	86	93
3	90	88
4	73	77
5	65	74
6	78	80
7	86	95
8	82	80
9	87	87
10	72	65

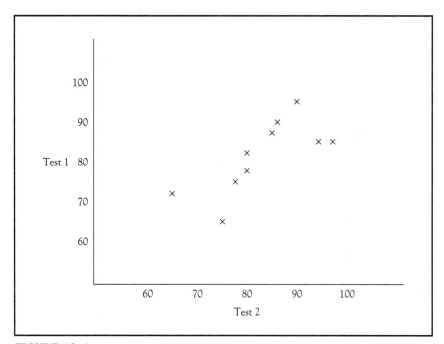

FIGURE 13–1. Scatter plot of speech discrimination test scores.

proportion of the total variance of the scores attributable to covariance, the higher the correlation. In the calculation of the correlation, the estimate of covariance is divided by the estimate of within-test variance.

In the present example, $r = .81$, indicating a strong relationship between the two tests. The proportion of total variance attributable to covariance is determined by squaring the correlation coefficient. When $r = .81$, $r^2 = 66$. This indicates the amount of variance that the two tests have in common. In this example, 66% of the variance in the scores of each test is related to the variance of the other test. To this extent, they are both measuring the same thing.

The correlation coefficient indicates the degree of relationship, but does not demonstrate that the correlation could not have occurred by chance. The statistical significance of the correlations, like the statistical significance of differences between measures, is expressed in terms of the .05 or .01 level of confidence. The significance depends on the size of the correlation and the number of subjects. If there are only 5 subjects, a correlation coefficient has to be .878 to be significant at the .05 level and .959 to be significant at the .01 level. If there are 100 subjects, the coefficient only has to be .195 for the .05 level and .254 for the .01 level. For the example in Table 13–1 and Figure 13–1, a correlation of .81 for 10 subjects would be significant beyond the .01 level.

If two variables were perfectly correlated, the scores would fall along a diagonal line, as in Figure 13–2. The correlation coefficients would approach 1.0 or -1.00, and r^2 would approach 100%, demonstrating that the two variables are perfectly related.

If there were no relationship between the scores on the two tests, the scatter plot would show an equal distribution of scores (see Figure 13–3).

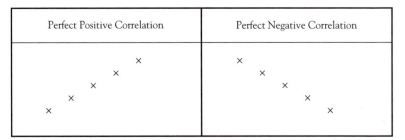

FIGURE 13–2. Hypothetical scatter plots showing a perfect positive correlation and a perfect negative correlation.

With such a perfect lack of correlation, both r and r^2 would approach .00. All of the variance would be attributable to variance within each set of measures, and none to covariance of the measures. The two measures could be said to be *independent*. However, conclusions concerning the independence of two variables on the basis of nonsignificant correlations greater than .00 should be made with extreme caution.

Low correlations can be interpreted only as indications of the independence of variables when both variables are adequately distributed. If there are ceiling or floor effects (see Chapter 9), as in the following extreme examples, correlations will be low because one variable is relatively invariant. In such cases, it would be wrong to conclude that the variables are independent (see Figure 13–4). If there is a ceiling or floor effect, any relationship that might exist is decreased by the upper or lower limit of the distribution. If there are ceiling effects, a more difficult test is needed to reach conclusions about the independence of variables, and if there are floor effects, an easier test is needed. This is one of the reasons why the distribution of scores should always be examined in interpreting HCD research.

Interpretation of Simple Correlations

Simple correlations can be interpreted in several ways, depending on the purpose of the research. In the above example, the correlation between

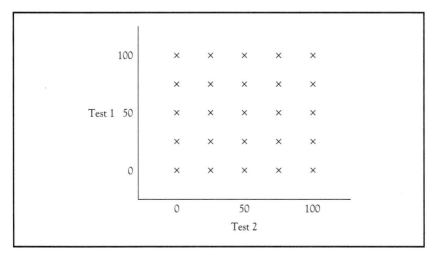

FIGURE 13–3.   Hypothetical scatter plots of uncorrelated variables.

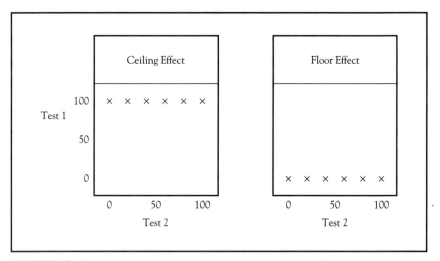

FIGURE 13–4. Hypothetical scatter plots showing a ceiling effect where all scores are maximum and a floor effect where all scores are at a minimum.

alternate forms of a speech discrimination test could serve as an index of the *reliability* of the test. If one is given in the clinic and the other test is given under real-life listening conditions, the correlation can serve as index of the *external validity* of the clinic test in predicting speech discrimination in real-life situations.

Whatever the interpretation of correlations, they apply only to the sample of subjects for whom the measures were obtained. For correlations as well as group designs, generalizing the results for a given sample of subjects to the entire population from which the sample was obtained is problematic. The recommended procedure is to *replicate* the findings by determining the correlation between measures for another group of subjects.

If the correlations involve a measure with questionable validity, such as a test of syntactic ability, it is also useful to estimate the extent to which the findings generalize to another measure of the same ability. This can be done by determining the correlation between the measure in question and another measure of the same ability, preferably a measure that has external validity. For example, scores on a syntax test might be correlated with the correctness of syntax in everyday conversations.

Simple correlations can be very useful for prediction, and also as tools for estimating the reliability and validity of measures. The main precaution regarding the interpretation of correlations is that they should not be taken at face value. It is advisable to replicate the findings with different subjects and different measures before making practical use of the findings. The samples should always be as large as possible. Small samples are not very informative. These precautions apply to all correlational procedures.

Other Tests of Simple Correlations

As with other parametric tests, certain assumptions are made for the Pearson product moment correlation test. The scores have to be evenly distributed, and the relationship between measures has to be *linear*. To be linear, the trend of the scatter plot has to be a straight line rather than a curved line. If these two assumptions are not met, the correlation coefficient may not give a valid indication of the relationship between measures.

Nonparametric tests of correlation avoid problems of distribution and linearity. A common nonparametric test for simple correlations is the *Spearman rank difference correlation*. The scores for each variable are ranked. The correlation coefficient, which is called *Rho* or *R*, is calculated on the basis of the difference between ranks. The smaller the differences between the pairs of ranks, the higher the correlation. If each subject's ranks tend to be the same for both measures, there will be small differences and a high positive correlation. High negative correlations occur when a high rank on one measure tends to be accompanied by a low rank on the other measure. Because of the conversion of scores to ranks, the nonparametric test is less powerful than the Pearson product moment test.

Point biserial correlation determines the relationship between two variables when one variable is divided into two categories and the other is normally distributed. An example would be the relationship between age and a pass or fail score on a clinical test. The *Phi coefficient* determines the relationship between two variables when both are scored in only two categories, such as pass and fail. Because of the conversion of scores to categories, these tests are less powerful than the Spearman rank difference test.

Intercorrelations Among Three or More Variables

A major limitation in the information obtained by correlation designs is that the correlation between two variables may be attributable to their joint correlations with other variables. This prevents any definite conclusions about the effect of one variable on the other. The same limitation applies to group designs that attempt to prove that a change in a dependent variable was caused by the independent variable and not by an uncontrolled variable.

An obvious way to determine the effects of uncontrolled variables is to calculate correlations between all relevant variables. Unfortunately, the intercorrelations among all relevant variables do not provide enough information by themselves. More complex correlational analyses are needed to assess the relationships among relevant variables. These analyses will be described in the following sections. In the early stages of research, however, it may be of interest to examine the intercorrelations in order to suggest the direction of further research. For example, if relevant uncontrolled variables such as age and education are found to be correlated with the variables that are being studied, such as syntactic ability, researchers know that the variables must be controlled in further research.

PARTIAL CORRELATION

When two variables are found to be correlated, it is often necessary to rule out the possibility that the relationship is attributable to their joint correlation with a third variable. The effect of the third variable can be "partialed out" by a very simple procedure called *partial correlation*. For example, there are three variables called A, B, and C, and the researchers are interested in the relationship between A (e.g., age) and B (e.g., amount of improvement in speechreading with 16 hours of training) independent of their joint relationship with C (amount of hearing loss). The correlations between A and B, A and C, and B and C are calculated. Then a simple formula is used to adjust the correlation between A and B to eliminate the influence of their joint correlation with C.

If there is a high negative correlation (e.g., $-.90$) between age (A) and amount of improvement with speechreading training (B), the researchers might conclude that learning ability decreases as a function of age. However, the relationship of age and improvement might be attributable to their joint correlation with amount of hearing loss (C). If the joint correlations are also high (e.g., .90 between age and hearing loss and $-.90$ between amount of improvement and hearing loss), removing their effects by partial correlation will greatly reduce the correlation between improvement and age (from $-.90$ to $-.47$) and the amount of common variance will be greatly reduced (from 81% to 22%). If the joint correlations are lower (e.g., .70 and −.70), the reduction in the correlation (−.90 to −.80) and in the common variance (81% to 64%) is not as great.

Partial correlation seems to be a very useful technique for estimating the unique relationship between two variables. In the previous example, other correlated variables such as visual acuity could also be partialed out to approach a causal explanation of the relationship between age and improvement with training. Some of the complex correlational procedures that will be described use a form of partial correlation to estimate unique relationships between variables.

As with all correlational procedures, however, partial correlations may be difficult to interpret. In the present example, it is not easy to determine which should be the relationship of interest. It may be as important to determine the relation of hearing loss to improvement with training as it is to determine the relationship between age and improvement. It is easy to become very confused. Partial correlations should be used only when the exact purpose is clear.

The information sought from partial correlations might also be obtained from a complex group design with age, amount of hearing loss, and amount of training as independent variables. Then the interrelationship among variables could be interpreted in terms of the interaction of Age × Hearing Loss × Training. Thus, the same problem could be investigated by using two different types of design. The choice of design would depend on the exact purpose of the research plus practical considerations such as the number and type of available subjects. Yet another way of approaching this particular problem would be to use analysis of covariance, a design that combines group and correlation designs; this design is described in a later section of this chapter.

MULTIPLE CORRELATION

Instead of being interested in the relationship between two variables, researchers may wish to determine the relationship of one variable (e.g., amount of improvement with auditory training) to a number of other variables (e.g., age, hearing impairment, education). *Multiple correlation* is a procedure for calculating the correlation between one variable and two or more other variables. The single variable is called the *criterion variable*, and can be considered the dependent variable. The multiple variables are called *predictor variables* and can be considered independent variables. Instead of partialing out the separate correlations of each predictor variable with the criterion variable, the joint relationship between the predictor (independent) variables and the criterion (dependent) variable is calculated.

In the examples used for partial correlation, it was of interest to evaluate the relationship between age and improvement when the effects of hearing loss had been removed. If the purpose had been to use all possible variables to help predict amount of success in speechreading training, a high correlation (e.g., −.90) between amount of improvement and age might have been sufficient by itself. If, however, there had been a lower correlation (e.g., −.70) between age and amount of improvement, other predictor variables might have been sought. Additional predictor variables will increase the correlation to the extent that their correlation with the criterion variable is high, and their correlations with the other predictor variables are low. If hearing loss is also correlated −.70 with improvement, the multiple correlation increases from −.70 (49% common variance) to −.81 (65% percent common variance) when the second predictor variable (hearing loss) is correlated .50 with the first predictor variable (age). The multiple correlation only increases from .70 to .77 (59% common variance) when the second predictor variable is correlated .70 with the first predictor variable. Additional predictor variables will increase the multiple correlation to the extent that they are highly correlated with the criterion variable and are not highly correlated with the other predictor variables.

Multiple correlations can be of practical value if they improve the prediction of the criterion variable for the subjects studied in the research, and if the predictions are equally good when the study is replicated with another sample of subjects. If the purpose is to get the best possible prediction of a criterion variable, multiple correlations can be very useful.

MULTIPLE REGRESSION

Multiple correlation improves predictions by combining the predictive power of several variables. However, it does not provide information about the separate contribution of each variable. Several procedures based on multiple correlation do provide such information. They are called *multiple regression* techniques. If used and interpreted with suitable caution, they have a great deal of potential value for problems for which group designs are inappropriate.

There are three main types of multiple regression. *Standard multiple regression* determines how much of the relationship between a set of predictor variables and a criterion variable is *uniquely* contributed by each of the predictor variables. For example, how much do each of the predictor variables of age and amount of hearing impairment contribute uniquely to the prediction of the amount of improvement with speechreading training? Such information could be very useful in assignments to groups for speechreading training, and in planning the total amount of training required for all groups. As discussed in connection with multiple correlation, the more highly intercorrelated the predictor variables, the lower their unique contribution.

A second type of multiple regression is *hierarchical regression*, in which the amount that a new predictor variable contributes to a multiple correlation is determined. For example, researchers might want to know if a speechreading aptitude test score would add substantially to the prediction of improvement with speechreading training. The multiple correlation of age and hearing loss with amount of improvement would be determined, and then the amount of change in the multiple correlation after the aptitude test score was added as a third predictor variable would be determined. This procedure would be of practical use in determining whether the time and expense involved in estimating aptitude would be of sufficient predictive value in planning training programs.

The third type of multiple regression is *stepwise regression*. For a given set of predictor variables, what is the order in which to enter predictor variables into the multiple regression equation for the best prediction of the criterion variable? This is another way to select the best set of predictor variables and to discard variables that do not contribute to the prediction.

Great care must be taken in using and interpreting multiple regression analyses. How much a given predictor variable contributes depends on its correlation with the other predictor variables. Preliminary research is helpful in selecting a useful set of predictors. Once the amount of predictive value of individual variables has been determined for one sample, a *replication* or *cross-validation* study should be carried out to determine whether the same results will be obtained with another sample. The ideal minimum number of subjects is 20 per predictor variable, and 10 subjects per variable is the practical minimum. The smaller the number of subjects, the greater the probability of overestimating the prediction. The need for large groups and for cross-validation is greatest for stepwise regression.

FACTOR ANALYSIS

If measures of a large number of variables have been obtained for a group of subjects, they may be grouped into subsets of highly correlated variables called *factors* by *factor analysis*. First, the intercorrelations among all the measures are calculated, and then the intercorrelations are mathematically "rotated" to group the most highly correlated measures into factors. Several different methods of factor analysis are available.

Factor analysis can be used to reduce the number of variables to be employed in further data analyses. For example, a number of language tests were administered to a group of subjects with language disorders, and three factors were found by factor analysis. The first factor included tests of word knowledge, the second tests of syntactic knowledge, and the third tests of discourse knowledge. For further research, the researchers could select the test that had the highest *factor loading*, that is, was most highly correlated with each factor. This would reduce the number of tests in the language test battery. Another procedure would be to use the *factor score* that was calculated for each factor as a composite score that best represented each factor. However, all of the original tests would have to be given to obtain the factor scores.

Great care must be taken in using and interpreting factor analysis. Factors are abstract entities and should not be interpreted as actual abilities. The factors obtained depend on the variables included and on the characteristics of the sample of subjects. Preliminary research is recommended to select measures, and cross-validation is recommended to confirm the findings with another sample. A major obstacle is the requirement for large samples of subjects. Factor analyses usually involve at least 10 variables, which would require minimum samples of 100 to 200 subjects.

Q FACTOR ANALYSIS AND CLUSTER ANALYSIS

The most common type of factor analysis, R *factor analysis*, groups variables into factors on the basis of the intercorrelations among the variables for a group of subjects. Q *factor analysis* groups subjects rather than tests into factors. The subjects are grouped into factors on the basis of similar patterns of test scores. If a number of tests of different language abilities were given to children with language disorders, and a Q factor analysis carried out, one factor might include subjects with especially low scores on language comprehension and another factor might include subjects with low scores on language expression. With this technique, then, subjects might be classified into subtypes of HCDs.

Cluster analysis also groups subjects into subgroups on the basis of similar patterns of scores, but with a different statistical technique. There are a number of different methods for cluster analysis, and it is important to determine which is most appropriate for a particular problem.

Q factor analysis and cluster analysis are promising methods for identifying different types of HCDs. They use a different approach from that of group designs to determine the characteristics of HCDs. Instead of assigning subjects to groups and then determining their characteristics, Q factor analysis and cluster analysis begin with an unselected group of subjects and statistically classify them into subgroups with similar characteristics. However, the usual cautions apply to the interpretation of these analyses. The factors and the clusters are abstract entities, not actual subtypes of disorders. The factors and clusters that are found depend on the variables assessed and the characteristics of the samples of subjects, as well as the particular statistical technique used. Within each factor or cluster, there may be considerable variability in the profiles of subjects.

ANALYSIS OF COVARIANCE

When a variable such as age needs to be controlled in a standard group design, the groups can be matched in age, or age can be systematically varied as one of the independent variables. If the variable cannot be controlled in this manner, a statistical control procedure called *analysis of covariance* or ANCOVA can be used. The groups being compared are equated for the uncontrolled variable by a technique that adjusts the means in a manner similar to partial correlation.

ANCOVA can serve three purposes. It can increase the power of the statistical tests of the effects of independent variables by removing the within-group variance attributable to the uncontrolled variable; it can statistically match the groups for the uncontrolled variable; and it can isolate the effects on multiple dependent variables in multivariate analysis of variance. ANCOVA can be a very useful tool for HCD research when relevant variables cannot be controlled because it permits valid group comparisons and increases statistical power. However, the adjusted means must be interpreted with caution, as with partial correlations.

MULTIVARIATE ANALYSIS OF VARIANCE

In some research, it may be of interest to have more than one dependent variable. For example, in studying the effects of therapy for voice disorders, researchers may wish to use both listener judgments and acoustic measures of voice quality before and after treatment. Both dependent variables can be analyzed by a single statistical procedure called *multivariate analysis of variance* or MANOVA. The two or more dependent variables are combined in such a way that they maximize differences between means for the main effects and interactions.

MANOVA serves several purposes. Error terms are chosen to adjust for the increased probability of chance differences with two or more dependent variables. The multivariate measure of combined dependent variables may provide a more sensitive test of the effects of the independent variable than would the separate dependent variables. Then the effects of the independent variables on each of the dependent variables separately can be determined by a procedure called *stepdown analysis*, in which the dependent variables are tested in a series of ANCOVAs by a method similar to hierarchical analysis in multiple regression.

MANOVA can be useful in the early stages of research, when researchers are not yet certain as to the most appropriate dependent variables to use for a particular problem. If variables are uncontrolled, MANOVA can be combined with ANCOVA to produce MANCOVA, the most complex variation of ANOVA. Because of the increase of complexity and the possible difficulty of interpretation, however, researchers should try to select a single dependent variable that will be most sensitive to the effects of the independent variables.

DISCRIMINANT ANALYSIS

The final technique that combines group and correlational designs is *discriminant function analysis*, usually called *discriminant analysis*. The basic technique is identical to that for a simple MANOVA for independent groups. Two or more dependent variables are combined in such a way that they maximally discriminate between two or more groups. Discriminant analysis is usually used to discriminate natural groups. The dependent variables can be considered predictor variables and the group classifications criterion variables.

For example, researchers may wish to predict the occurrence of language disorders at age 4 on the basis of language and nonlanguage tests given to a sample of at-risk 2-year-olds. When the subjects have been classified into groups with and without language disorders on the basis of their language ability at age 4, a discriminant analysis would determine the weighted combination of the 2-year-old scores that best discriminates the groups. Then a weighted score can be calculated for each child, and the distributions of scores for the two groups can be compared to determine the amount of overlap in scores. If the dependent variables are not highly correlated, the group distributions may not overlap at all even though the distributions for each of the predictor variables do overlap. In such a case, the weighted scores for 2-year-olds can be used to predict whether they will have a language disorder at age 4.

Discriminant analysis can be very useful for maximizing the accuracy of diagnosing HCDs. Like all other correlational procedures, however, discriminant analyses must be interpreted with caution, and no causal inferences can be made on the basis of discriminant analysis alone. There should be at least twice as many subjects in each group as there are dependent variables, with a minimum of 20 per group if at all possible. If it is necessary to reduce the number of variables to accommodate small groups, multiple stepwise regression can be used to eliminate variables that contribute the least to the prediction. Cross-validation with another sample of subjects should be carried out to confirm the weighting of scores.

ADDITIONAL INFORMATION

Additional information about the statistical analyses of relationships is given in the following texts:

Afifi, A. A., & Clark, V. (1990). *Computer-aided multivariate analysis* (2nd ed.). New York: Van Nostrand & Rheinhold.

Childs, D. (1990). *The essentials of factor analysis* (2nd ed.). London: Cassell Educational.

Everitt, B. S. (1993). *Cluster analysis* (3rd ed.). New York: Halsted.

Everitt, B. S., & Dunn, G. (1992). *Applied multivariate data analysis.* New York: Oxford University Press.

Stevens, J. (1992). *Applied multivariate statistics for the social sciences* (2nd ed.). Hillsdale, NJ: Erlbaum.

✦ ✦ ✦ ✦ ✦ ✦ ✦ REVIEW QUESTIONS ✦ ✦ ✦ ✦ ✦ ✦ ✦

1. Define the terms *covariance* and *regression*.

2. Give examples of high positive correlations and high negative correlations.

3. How are correlations used for predictions?

4. Create several sets of data involving 10 pairs of scores and make a scatter plot for each set. Try to make examples of high positive correlations, high negative correlations, and low correlations.

5. What information is obtained by squaring the correlation coefficient?

6. What do ceiling and floor effects do to correlations?

7. How are correlations used to demonstrate reliability and validity?

8. What information is needed to calculate a partial correlation?

9. What is the difference between partial and multiple correlation?

10. Describe the three types of multiple regression.

11. What is meant by factor loadings and factor scores?

12. How do Q factor analysis and cluster analysis differ from R factor analysis?

13. What are the three purposes for using ANCOVA?

14. What are the advantages and disadvantages of MANOVA?

15. What are the advantages and disadvantages of discriminant analysis?

Interpretation
of Research

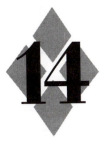

Interpretation is the culmination of the research. After the data have been collected and analyzed, the researchers have to evaluate the findings. If a study had very specific and very limited goals, the interpretation may involve a simple list of the findings. In most HCD research, however, different aspects of the research are examined to reach conclusions concerning the amount and type of new knowledge.

The exact manner of interpretation depends on the aspect of HCDs studied and the purpose. There may be as many as six stages of interpretation:

1. Have the findings accomplished the purpose?

2. What limitations are placed on the interpretation by the design, procedure, and method of analysis?

3. How does the new knowledge relate to previous knowledge concerning the problem?

4. Can practical applications be recommended?

5. What further research is needed?

6. What final conclusions can be drawn?

The first three stages are usually included, but not necessarily in the order given here. Recommendations for practical applications and suggestions for further research may or may not be offered, and there may not be a final conclusion. As is the case for other research events, HCD researchers tailor the interpretation to meet the needs of their research.

The stages of interpretation can be illustrated by the hypothetical study of the benefits of training in speechreading used as an example for the factorial ANOVA in Chapter 12.

ACCOMPLISHMENT OF THE ORIGINAL PURPOSE

The purpose states what the researchers wish to find. The statement may be in the form of questions, hypotheses derived from a theory, or predictions based on past knowledge. As a first step in the interpretation of findings, the researchers decide whether the purpose was accomplished. In the study of speechreading training, the purpose was to determine the benefits of training for younger and older persons with acquired sensorineural hearing loss. The purpose could have been stated as questions: Will speechreading continue to improve as more training is given? Will younger persons benefit more than older persons? Or as predictions: There should be steady improvement with training, and younger persons should improve more.

Evaluation of the findings in relation to the purpose would reveal that there was steady improvement in speechreading with training, and that younger subjects improved more. The basic findings can be stated in a clear and simple manner. This initial interpretation does not go beyond the immediate findings. Further interpretations are made in the later stages.

LIMITATIONS IMPOSED BY THE DESIGN, PROCEDURE, AND ANALYSIS

The evaluation of results in terms of the inherent limitations of the research events is a crucial point in the research. The researchers have done their best to fill an important gap in knowledge, and must now decide just what they have found. Their interpretation is limited by their own research events. They cannot draw conclusions about independent variables that were not varied, dependent variables that were not measured, and populations of subjects that were not sampled. Their conclusions are also limited by the exact procedures and methods of data analysis that were used.

Before the researchers decide on their contribution to knowledge, the limitations imposed by the design, procedure, and analysis must be reviewed. What independent variables were identified for study? Were relevant variables adequately controlled? To what extent did the study have internal and external validity? Were the dependent variables measured in a reliable manner? How large and representative were the samples of subjects? Were the procedures adequately defined and properly carried out? What kind of information was yielded by the data analyses? The entire machinery of the study may be reexamined. In most HCD research, compromises must be made in the ideal requirements for design, procedure, and analysis because of practical considerations. The effects of these compromises are considered at this stage of interpretation.

In the study of training in speechreading, specific amounts of training of a particular type were given to particular samples of younger and older subjects. Their progress was assessed by a particular test of word recognition, and the findings were analyzed by a particular statistical technique. The study was a relatively simple comparison of three different amounts of training with two different groups. In interpreting the results, the researchers should confirm that relevant variables were controlled. If unmatched groups had been used, the advantage of younger subjects might have been attributable to the tendency for younger subjects to have more education and less hearing loss. Training conditions should have been the same for both groups, with enough preliminary instruction and practice that older subjects would not be penalized. There should have been some basis for estimating whether the word recognition task predicted speechreading ability in natural situations. The effects of the ceiling effect for the younger subjects after 16 hours of training should have been carefully considered. Conclusions concerning the benefits of training should have been applied only to the specific training procedure that was used. Other aspects of the design, procedure, and analysis that might have affected the findings, such as the reliability of judging spoken responses, also should have been examined.

The extent to which limitations must be discussed depends on the characteristics of the study. If age, gender, education, hearing loss, cultural background, type of training, and longer periods of training had been included as independent variables, and both performance on a word recognition test and evaluation in a natural setting as dependent variables, the interpretation would be less limited. In a relatively modest study like the one cited here, in which there were only two independent variables, one dependent variable, and small groups, the researchers' interpretation would be limited to the suggestion that training of a particular type and duration might have more benefits for younger subjects.

RELATION TO PREVIOUS KNOWLEDGE

Researchers review previous knowledge to determine how much is already known or guessed about a problem. After the research is carried out, they must decide whether their findings confirm, contradict, or add new information to previous theories and research.

A review of previous knowledge about the benefits of training in speechreading might have revealed more informed guesswork than knowledge gained through research. There might be skepticism about the benefits of formal training, especially training in the recognition of visual cues for isolated speech sounds. The small amount of previous research might suggest some benefits for formal training, but be generally inconclusive. Within such a framework of previous knowledge, the findings might confirm the benefits of training and provide new information about the effects of age.

If the findings add a small, definite amount of new information, comparisons with previous research can be brief and concise. If the findings are more complex, a detailed comparison of the design, procedure, and analysis of the past and present research may be necessary. For the present example, a fairly narrow interpretation in relation to previous research might be sufficient. Previous findings concerning the benefits of training in speechreading are supported and extended. Research on the same topic using different approaches might be more controversial and require much more extensive interpretation in relation to previous knowledge.

PRACTICAL APPLICATIONS

The possibility of practical applications of research findings depends on how definite the findings are relative to the theories used by practitioners. If practice is based largely on informed guesswork and there is no potential danger in applying findings, researchers may suggest the possible benefit of practical applications. This might occur if there is a valid and reliable demonstration that a new approach is superior to a practical approach based largely on guesswork.

Before making such suggestions, the researchers must review previous knowledge and specify the limitations imposed by the design, procedure, and analysis. In the present example, it might be suggested that practitioners who had not found a highly successful procedure for training speechreading could try some variation of the procedure used in the study. However, suitable cautions would be necessary regarding the small, restricted samples of subjects; the limited subject and task variables assessed; the single type of training; the limited amount of training; the single dependent variable; and the ceiling effect that limited the data analysis.

Suggestions for practical applications vary widely with the types of HCDs and the aspects of HCDs studied. In the majority of research, suggestions are made very cautiously, and are often accompanied by statements that further research is required for more definite recommendations.

FURTHER RESEARCH

As a direct consequence of assessing the limitations of their findings, relating the findings to previous knowledge, and deciding on practical suggestions, researchers can suggest what further research might be needed. This is another crucial point in research. The researchers have done their best to formulate and carry out research on an important problem and have realistically appraised their findings. They are in a very good position to make specific suggestions about the further research needed to obtain useful information about the problem. At this point in the interpretation, additional results such as descriptive statistics, data for individual subjects, and qualitative data of various kinds might be useful in suggesting the direction of further research.

In some cases, no further information may be needed regarding the specific topic of research. In others, the results might point to the need for further studies of the same type, using additional independent and dependent variables to add systematically to the information provided by the first study. If the findings have been sufficiently inconclusive, a completely different research approach might be suggested. If knowledge about a problem can be provided only by a series of studies, suggestions regarding further research are of the greatest importance.

In the study of speechreading training, if the limited findings were interpreted as suggesting the usefulness of training, and present knowledge was considered inadequate, a series of studies could be suggested. Samples of subjects of different ages, genders, levels of education, degrees of hearing loss, and cultural backgrounds could be selected. Different types of training could be designed. Larger amounts of training could be given. Results could be assessed with several different dependent variables, with long-term follow-up. If there was a question about the usefulness of speechreading training, research could be designed to compare speechreading training with other rehabilitation strategies. Different types of research design, such as qualitative methods (Chapter 18) might be suggested for such research. All of these suggestions would be made with the practical goals of HCD research in mind.

CONCLUSIONS

In drawing final conclusions, researchers can speculate in general terms about the implications of their findings and the current state of knowledge about the problem. Examination of research reports in the *Journal of Speech and Hearing Research* suggests that final conclusions may restate the main findings, recommend practical applications, or suggest further research. HCD researchers do not lose sight of their goals, and they draw conclusions on the basis of a careful interpretation of what they have found in relation to past knowledge. If they feel confident of their findings, they present them as new knowledge, and if the findings seem suitable in relation to present practices, they make recommendations for practical applications. If knowledge is still incomplete, they suggest the types of further research that are needed. The concluding statement completes the contribution to knowledge for this particular research. If the researchers feel that the topic is important enough to pursue, they will plan and carry out more research.

ADDITIONAL INFORMATION

The interpretation of findings is discussed in the books on research methods cited at the end of Chapters 1 and 3.

• • • • • • • • REVIEW QUESTIONS • • • • • • • •

1. List the six stages that may be included in the interpretation of HCD research, and briefly describe each.

2. For a current issue of the *Journal of Speech and Hearing Research*, list the stages of interpretation that are included. Interpretations are found in sections headed Discussion, Conclusions, and Results and Discussion.

PART II

Other Research Methods

The standard group research methods described in Part I provide researchers with tools that, if used with suitable caution, can yield useful information about HCDs. There is a well-established logic behind these methods that allows researchers to arrive at valid, if sometimes limited, conclusions about the phenomena they study. However, as discussed in Chapter 7, these methods are far from perfect. Some of the other research methods presented in this section represent attempts to overcome the disadvantages of standard group methods.

Observational and descriptive methods (Chapter 15) provide quantitative and qualitative descriptions of individuals and groups and can supplement the information obtained by other methods. Single subject methods (Chapter 17) and case study methods (Chapter 15) provide information about individual subjects. Single subject methods and path analysis (Chapter 19) are methods for studying cause-and-effect relationships. Qualitative methods (Chapter 18) provide a means for going beyond quantitative information. Statistical power analysis (Chapter 19) overcomes limitations of the null hypothesis. Meta-analysis and multiple methods (Chapter 16) base conclusions on multiple sources of data. Path analysis and maximum likelihood estimation (Chapter 19) test theoretical models; and maximum likelihood estimation provides information about both individuals and groups. Loglinear methods (Chapter 19) analyze multidimensional categorical data; and sequential analysis enables researchers to study the contingencies involved in communicative interactions.

These methods are alternative tools available to HCD researchers. They can be extremely useful in overcoming the limitations of standard group research methods. However, each has its own inherent limitations. There is no such thing as a perfect research method. It is important to note that standard group methods serve HCD research very well. Of the 104 studies published in the *Journal of Speech and Hearing Research* in 1994, 91 used the standard group methods described in Part I.

Observational, Case Study, and Descriptive Methods

The three methods discussed in this chapter have been used as long or longer than the standard group methods described in Part I. They all differ from the standard group methods in that they do not involve inferential statistical analysis. It should be noted, however, that observational methods can be used for data collection and descriptive methods for data reduction in research using standard group methods.

OBSERVATION IN NATURAL SETTINGS

Observational methods are used to obtain quantitative or qualitative information in natural settings. The use of observational methods to obtain quantitative information will be discussed here, and the use of these methods to obtain qualitative information will be discussed in Chapter 18.

The main difference between observational methods and standard group designs is that in the former there is no attempt to control all relevant variables in order to isolate the effects of independent variables. However, observational methods should not be confused with the casual observations made in everyday life. The behaviors to be observed are defined in advance, and the observations are carefully recorded.

Recording is done by videotape or audiotape, by notes made by observers, or by tallies of observed behaviors made by the observers. The objective is to identify behaviors and relationships among behaviors in natural contexts. In some cases, it is the effect of the context that is being studied. Several types of observation will be briefly described as related to HCD research.

Observation Without Intervention

In *observation without intervention*, passive observers simply record the events that occur in natural settings. These methods are also called *naturalistic observation*. In HCD research, naturalistic observation can be used to verify relationships among variables found by the use of standard group designs. For example, HCD and non-HCD subjects could be observed in natural settings to verify differences in characteristics such as misarticulation, voice disorders, or nonfluency, and to determine whether prior intervention has resulted in improved communication in natural settings. Naturalistic observation can also be used to determine the effects of different contexts on HCDs, for example, whether the rate of dysfluency varies in home, school, recreational, and vocational settings.

Observation with Intervention

To obtain particular types of information, observers may intervene in several different ways. In *participant observation*, the observer becomes a participant in the situation in order to understand the situation of the person observed. This method is better suited to qualitative than to quantitative research. In *structured observation*, the observers control the situation in certain ways to obtain the desired information. A child with language disorder and a child without language disorder may be put in a play situation with specially selected toys to provide information about the communicative interactions of children with language disorders in natural settings. More situational control is exerted in *field experiments*, in which an elaborate situation may be "staged" to determine its effects on participants. Stutterers might be asked to participate in situations in which the other participants have been trained to exhibit anger, impatience, scorn, and sympathy to determine the effects of such social stresses on dysfluency.

Communicative Interactions

A type of structured observation that is used very often in HCD research is the observation of communicative interactions in natural settings. The communicative interactions usually involve various combinations of children with and without HCDs, and children interacting with adults. These structured observations often provide the best way of obtaining the desired information about the effects of HCDs. What is observed is an interaction between two or more subjects, not the response of a subject to a controlled stimulus. The researchers usually attempt to reach conclusions concerning the HCDs of one of the participants. In most cases, the basic data are units of communicative behavior such as demands, questions, requests for action, and comments. These data can be quantified in terms of relative frequency and duration, and can be rated on subjective dimensions. Sequential patterns of responses can also be quantified, such as the relative frequency of different responses to requests for action. Situational comparisons can be made, such as the relative frequency of verbal and nonverbal communicative responses in the interaction of a child with HCD and a child without HCD as compared with the interaction of 2 children with HCD.

Advantages and Disadvantages of Observational Methods

Observational methods involve situations much closer to real-life settings and clinic settings. They provide detailed, ecologically valid information that cannot be obtained in any other way. However, the information obtained from observation of individuals in particular natural settings cannot easily be generalized to other individuals or to other settings, and the lack of systematic control of relevant variables precludes the provision of precise information about interactions, correlations, or causal relationships.

Problems that researchers must be particularly concerned with in natural observation are observer bias and subject bias. Researchers must rule out the possibility that observers will be unduly influenced by what they expect and hope to observe, and the possibility that the subjects will be unduly influenced by the knowledge that they are being observed.

CASE STUDIES

The classic method for obtaining detailed information about individuals with HCDs is the case study. The information can be obtained from a number of sources, including developmental history, medical history, home and educational background, clinical observations, test results, and responses to treatment. Case studies may be restricted to one individual with a rare disorder, or to a series of individuals with similar disorders. They can be used to supplement the information obtained from group designs. The case study method is especially appropriate for obtaining information about types of HCD that occur too rarely to be studied by the use of group designs. For example, there are relatively few deaf–blind individuals, but it is important to evaluate the effectiveness of communicative training with such individuals. This is best done by case studies.

Case studies provide evidence about individuals that is not usually intended to be generalized to a population. Therefore, formal methods of statistical analysis are unnecessary. The data are quantitative and qualitative descriptions of representative cases of a particular HCD, a rare disorder, or a new treatment. Descriptions may be relatively brief or fairly detailed, sometimes book length. A great deal of the value of the case study depends on the researchers' ability to select and highlight relevant information and to integrate the information in a logical manner in relation to previous knowledge.

A major advantage of case studies is that there is no restriction on the amount or type of information included. In addition, they can suggest directions for further research, can be used to study new techniques and rare phenomena, and can provide important tests for theories. The disadvantages are that it is difficult to generalize from a single case, that uncontrolled observations of individuals do not provide information about interactions, correlations, or causal relationships, and that there can be bias in the selection of cases, the selection of information about cases, and the interpretation of findings.

Researchers may do case studies when other designs are inappropriate, or when they want to obtain information for planning research that uses other designs. Conclusions from case studies are informed guesswork. Practitioners who keep detailed case histories concerning particularly informative cases can present their findings as case studies. Thus, the case study brings researchers and practitioners close together.

DESCRIPTIVE METHODS

Some writers classify observational methods and case study methods as *descriptive methods*. The term is used here to denote methods for gathering quantitative information that may include descriptive statistics, tables, and graphs, but not inferential statistics. The information may concern individuals or groups.

Individual Description

Some HCDs involve uniform physiological processes. When variability between individuals is small enough, group designs are unnecessary. Useful information can be obtained via observation of individuals under carefully controlled conditions. Examples would be studies of reflex responses of jaw, lip, and tongue muscles. If individual differences in uncontrolled variables do not confound the effects of independent variables, the findings of individual descriptive studies can be generalized to others in the same population. If the level of the independent variable is changed as part of the study, information can be obtained about causal relationships, as in the effect of cleft palate surgery on speech. For certain phenomena, then, the objectives of group designs can be achieved in studies of individuals. It is important for HCD researchers to be aware of this possibility, even though such phenomena may be relatively rare.

Group Description

HCD research sometimes involves very careful studies that do not determine the effects of independent variables, but simply describe variables of interest in a normal population or a population with HCDs. The information is obtained under the carefully controlled conditions that are required by standard group designs, but there is no experiment. The results are reported in detail to provide information about the range of variation in normal or HCD populations. For example, spontaneous speech samples might be obtained for a large sample of normal speakers to determine the incidence of dysfluencies in normal speech. Another example of group description designs would be surveys of a population by means of questionnaires. Surveys can reveal important information about the characteristics, attitudes, educational achievements, and case histories of large samples of HCDs. However, there may be questions about the reliability of self-reports.

ADDITIONAL INFORMATION

Observational Methods:

Shaughnessy, J. J., & Zechmeister, E. B. (1985). *Research methods in psychology.* New York: Knopf.

Sommer, B., & Sommer, R. (1991). *A practical guide to behavioral research* (3rd ed.). New York: Oxford University Press.

Case Studies:

Yin, R. K. (1994). *Case study research: Design and method.* Thousand Oaks, CA: Sage.

Yin, R. K. (1993). *Applications of case study research.* Newbury Park, CA: Sage.

Descriptive Methods (see also Shaughnessy & Zechmeister, 1985, above):

Foddy, W. (1993). *Constructing questions for interviews and questionnaires.* New York: Cambridge University Press.

Weisberg, H. F., Krosnick, J. A., & Bowen, B. D. (1989). *An introduction to survey research and data analysis* (2nd ed.). Glenview, IL: Scott, Foresman.

Wentland, E. J. (1993). *Survey responses: An evaluation of their validity.* San Diego: Academic Press.

Statistical Power Analysis, Meta-Analysis, and Multiple Methods

Acornerstone of the standard group research methods described in Part I is the null hypothesis. This method of proof has been criticized as not providing enough information about the *magnitude* of experimental effects. *Statistical power analysis* is a procedure for estimating the magnitude of experimental effects in terms of *effect size*, and *meta-analysis* is a procedure for estimating effect size for a group of studies. *Multiple methods* reduce problems of reliability and validity by obtaining multiple measures of the variables studied.

STATISTICAL POWER ANALYSIS

The *null hypothesis* is the accepted standard of proof in HCD and other behavioral sciences. As described in Chapter 10, a given significance level—usually the .05 or .01 level—is selected, and the null hypothesis is rejected if the statistical test yields a probability at or below this level. This method of proof gives the probability that the null hypothesis might be rejected if there is actually no difference or no relationship between the populations under study. It guards against a Type I error—concluding that there is a difference or relationship when there is none. Whether the .05 or the .01 level is selected depends on how much risk of a Type I error the researcher is prepared to make.

Although the null hypothesis provides a very conservative method of proof, it does not provide any information beyond the chances of a Type I error. Statistical power analysis (Cohen, 1988) provides more information about the magnitude of observed differences and relationships. The statistical power of a study is a function of the preselected significance level, the number of subjects in each group, and a third value—the *effect size*. For studies of differences between groups, the effect size is usually the standardized difference between means, as calculated by dividing the difference between means by the within-group standard deviation. For studies of relationships, the effect size is usually the correlation coefficient.

Statistical power is the probability that a statistical test will yield statistically significant results. This sounds almost like the null hypothesis, but it is not. The null hypothesis estimates the probability that there will be a statistically significant result when there is actually *no* difference or relationship in the populations studied. Statistical power analysis states the probability that a statistically significant difference or relationship will be found when there *is* a difference or relationship in the populations studied. As stated before, statistical power is a function of the significance level, the number of subjects, and the effect size. The larger the significance level, the number of subjects, and the effect size, the greater the statistical power.

Researchers can use statistical power analysis to evaluate the power of studies that have already been carried out and to plan studies that will have sufficient probability of yielding significant results. An example may be helpful. In a study of two groups of 30 subjects each, in which one group received treatment and the other did not, the significance level was set at .01, and the effect size (difference between means divided by standard deviation) was .5 (one half of a standard deviation), the statistical power of a *t*-test would be .24. This would indicate that there was only about a 25% chance, or one chance in four, for statistical significance. There are a number of ways in which the statistical power could be increased:

1. If the .05 level were selected instead of the .01 level, the statistical power would increase from .24 to .47, almost one chance in two of a significant result.

2. If the number of subjects per group were increased to 60, the statistical power at the .05 level would further increase to .77, or more than three chances in four of a significant effect.

3. If a one-tailed *t*-test were used (Chapter 11) instead of a two-tailed test at the .05 level, the statistical power would increase to .86, or about five chances in six of a significant result.

4. Finally, if the effect size were increased from .5 to .8, the statistical power of a one-tailed *t*-test at the .05 level for 60 subjects per group would increase to beyond 99%! Effect size could be increased either by increasing the difference between means or decreasing the within-group standard deviations. The difference between means might increase if more sessions of treatment were given or a different treatment was used, and the standard deviations might be decreased by carefully selecting subjects in terms of such variables as age, education, and severity of disorder.

As this example shows, researchers can use statistical power analysis to avoid designing studies in which there is little chance of significant findings.

Determination of Statistical Power and Sample Size

In the planning of research or evaluation of previous research, statistical power and sample size can be easily determined by the use of tables supplied by Cohen (1988). Tables are provided for *t*-tests, Pearson product moment correlations, differences between correlation coefficients, tests of proportions, chi-square tests, analysis of variance and covariance, multiple regression, and set correlation. In order to estimate statistical power, significance level, sample size, and effect size must be known. In order to estimate sample size, statistical power, significance level, and sample size must be known.

Other Considerations

Statistical power is not commonly reported in HCD research, although statistical power analysis may often be used in the planning of studies. Researchers should be familiar with power analysis because power analyses are often required in research grant applications. As time goes on, power analyses may also be required by journal editors and thesis examiners. Several microcomputer programs for power analyses are available (Cohen, 1988), including tutorials, and undoubtedly more will be supplied in future statistical packages.

One of the main applications of power analysis has been power surveys of research in psychology, education, medicine, sociology, and criminology. The results of these surveys have not been encouraging. Except for fields in which large numbers of subjects are readily available, the average power found in surveys did not usually exceed .5. In a survey of research in HCD, Kroll and Chase (1975) reported results very similar to those obtained in other fields. For small and medium effect sizes, statistical power was too low. In such a case, there would be too many Type II errors (failing to reject the null hypothesis when there was an experimental effect) relative to Type I errors. This led the authors to wonder how many studies have not been reported because the power was so low that the results were nonsignificant.

Power analysis should be part of researchers' strategy. It can be useful in planning research where the values chosen for significance level, number of subjects, effect size, and desired statistical power will also reflect considerations specific to the study, such as the availability of subjects. If there is no way to obtain adequate statistical power, the research could be carried out as a pilot study.

A major application of power analysis has been in meta-analysis, as described in the next section.

META-ANALYSIS

Surveys of research on a given topic, such as the effects of treatment on a particular HCD, are often presented in the form of review articles, in which the reviewer arrives at a judgment of the overall contribution to knowledge. The advent of statistical power analysis led to the development of a quantitative procedure called *meta-analysis*, designed for evaluating the evidence contained in multiple studies on the same topic. Meta-analysis is intended to overcome the shortcomings of individual studies and is considered less open to bias than traditional literature reviews. If so, meta-analyses can make an important contribution to cumulative knowledge.

Most research in the behavioral sciences has involved individual studies. In the physical sciences, methods for combining evidence from multiple studies have been used since the 1930s, and research centers that specialize in the systematic synthesis of information from multiple studies have been functioning for many years. About 20 years ago, the term *meta-*

analysis was applied to the evaluation of multiple studies in psychology and related disciplines. Now the results of many meta-analyses are published every year in psychology, psychiatry, education, and related disciplines.

Although there are several different quantitative approaches to meta-analysis, the basic idea is quite simple. The contribution to knowledge is evaluated in terms of some value related to the average effect size in the group of studies. It will be recalled that for studies of differences between groups, the effect size is usually the standardized difference between means, as calculated by dividing the difference between means by the within-group standard deviation; and for studies of relationships, the effect size is usually the correlation coefficient. Not only main effects such as treatment versus no treatment, but also the interactive effects of "moderator variables" such as age, education, severity of disorder, and type of treatment can be evaluated, provided that there are sufficient studies involving the moderator variables.

The complexities of meta-analysis relate to the exact procedures used to correct for "artifacts" such as measurement error, range restriction, and dichotomization of measures before calculating effect size. As meta-analytic techniques become more precise and more complex statistically, a great deal of special knowledge may be required to carry out and interpret the analyses (Schmidt, 1992). However, the applications of meta-analyses in HCD research may not be too demanding, and there is no shortage of books on how to do meta-analysis (e.g., Cooper & Hedges, 1994; Hunter & Schmidt, 1990; Rosenthal, 1991).

Meta-analyses involve many strategic decisions. Before the distribution of effect sizes can be plotted, there are a number of steps to be taken that require time, effort, and careful planning (Hattie & Hansford, 1984):

1. The first consideration is to select a topic. It should be in the researchers' field of expertise, unless they are collaborating with someone who has adequate knowledge about the topic. The topic should not have been the subject of a previous meta-analysis, unless the purpose is cross-validation. It is not always necessary to select a topic for which the findings of studies have been consistent and predictable, resulting in small variation of effect sizes. It may be just as interesting to study topics in which effect sizes are highly variable, and then determine the interacting moderator variables (such as type of treatment) that contribute to the variability.

2. The next step is to initiate a literature search. Literature searches using computerized databases such as PsycLit and Medline can be very

helpful. In most areas of HCD research, it should be possible to specify the journals that contain studies on the topic. If there are not too many, it may be possible to look through the journals themselves for the last few years. Such a procedure, if feasible, is preferable to relying exclusively on computer searches, which are far from infallible. References to previous research on the topic can be obtained from the most recent studies. It is advisable to photocopy the studies that are selected for meta-analysis.

3. Once the research reports have been selected, the information necessary for calculating "clean" estimates of effect size corrected for artifacts must be obtained. If information concerning means and standard deviations is not directly available, the researchers may have to be contacted.

4. A decision must be made as to what studies should be included. One meta-analysis of the aphasia treatment literature (Wachter & Straf, 1990) selected only 13 of 114 studies! Because the total number of available studies in many areas of HCD may be much smaller, the decision at this point might be whether there are enough studies to carry out a meta-analysis. If meta-analysis does not seem advisable and the topic is sufficiently important, a traditional review of the literature could be carried out with the studies that have been selected.

5. If the meta-analysis is to be carried out, a particular method of analysis has to be selected. Consultation with an expert may be necessary. The method selected will dictate the exact procedures for coding, correction for artifacts, differential weighting of studies, and other steps to be taken in calculating effect sizes. Microcomputer programs are available for aiding these computations.

6. The final step, as in all research, is interpreting the findings. For those unfamiliar with meta-analysis, a clear statement of the findings and the evaluation of the contribution to knowledge is needed. The conclusions may be tentative if there are relatively few studies, or the studies are of dubious quality. The results may point to the need for further research.

Advantages and Disadvantages

Proponents of meta-analysis (e.g., Schmidt, 1992) consider it not merely a way of combining the information contained in multiple studies, but also a major advance in cumulative knowledge. Individual studies are only single data points for future meta-analyses. Only meta-analyses can control chance and artifacts and provide a trustworthy foundation for conclusions. "Primary" researchers specialize in conducting individual studies, according to this view, and meta-analysts make the actual scientific discoveries.

There is no question that meta-analysis can be of great use for scientific discoveries, but, as is the case for all research methods, it must be applied with great caution. Sohn (1995) pointed out that meta-analysis is not based on the *direct* study of phenomena. Going from the primary data to meta-analysis entails potential pitfalls, especially considering the number of different methods of analysis. The quality of the studies on which meta-analyses are based may be questionable (Wachter & Straf, 1990). Moreover, in selecting studies to serve as data points, the meta-analysts do not have access to research that was never reported because the results were unpromising. The absence of such studies from the distribution of effect sizes can increase the chances of incorrectly rejecting the null hypothesis, that is, of making a Type I error.

Conclusions

HCD researchers should be generally familiar with meta-analysis, and also with any meta-analyses that have been carried out in their field of interest. In HCD research, for example, Robey (1994) analyzed the efficacy of treatment of aphasics, reporting on the basis of 21 studies "clear superiority" in the performance of aphasics receiving treatment by speech–language pathologists. Bat-Chava (1993) analyzed 42 studies of the antecedents of self-esteem in deaf people, reporting that self-esteem tended to be higher when parents were deaf and when sign language was used in the home.

Meta-analyses should be done by researchers who have compelling questions that might be answered by this method. The amount and type of work required for meta-analyses will not appeal to all researchers. Those who do meta-analyses should be serious students of the subject, knowledgeable about the techniques involved, aware of potential pitfalls, and able to view meta-analyses in the context of other strategies of HCD research. Great care is required at all stages. For example, in evaluating treatment studies, the exact method of treatment should be considered, as well as the nontreatment or alternative treatment control groups that were used (Eysenck, 1995). The quality of the studies in other respects must also be carefully considered; and the selection of studies must not be biased toward a particular theoretical viewpoint. HCD research is a potentially fruitful area for meta-analysis because there are important practical questions to be answered.

MULTIPLE METHODS

Multiple research methods have been recommended for many years. Meta-analysis as a method for analyzing multiple studies was discussed here, and triangulation will be mentioned as a method for using multiple sources of data in qualitative research in Chapter 18. Several other methods are briefly described here.

Multimethod Multitrait Matrix

Campbell and Fiske (1959) proposed a *multimethod multitrait matrix*, in which a number of different traits, such as verbal, spatial, and mathematical abilities, are each assessed by a number of different methods, such as standard tests, interviews, and course grades. This procedure enables the researchers to estimate the reliability and validity of the measures of the traits. The rationale behind this and other multiple methods is that no single measure can be a perfect measure of a process. Extraneous stimulus and response variables always contribute error variance. The multimethod multitrait matrix provides a model for planning research that will yield improved measures. Although this procedure has not been widely used, the idea behind it has been recognized as important; Campbell and Fiske's (1959) paper is one of the most often cited articles in the psychological literature.

Methodological Pluralism

Roth (1987) used the term *methodological pluralism* to describe the investigation of phenomena by completely different methods. In an interesting application of this method, Angus (1992) made an initial qualitative study of metaphor in psychotherapy and then designed a series of quantitative studies to explore correlates of metaphor identified in the qualitative analysis.

Critical Multiplism

Critical multiplism (Mark & Shotland, 1987; Shadish, 1986) involves the use of different investigators, locations, populations, implementations of independent variables, sites, outcome measures, statistical methods, data analysts, and theorists to study a particular problem. The term *critical* refers to the careful choice of the multiple aspects, as opposed to what is termed a *shotgun approach*. One preferred analytic approach for critical multiplism is causal modeling (see Chapter 19).

Multiple Case Research

Rosenwald (1988) proposed a quite different multiple method. In his model of *multiple case research*, a small number of individuals are intensively interviewed over a period of time and brought into "conversation" with one another by means of the researchers' qualitative analysis. Discrepant images about shared realities are reconstructed to arrive at a *socialization of viewpoints*. The method recognizes that unique personalities cannot be averaged across individuals and provides a way of demonstrating how personality is shaped by social interaction.

Conclusions

Despite their advantages in overcoming problems of reliability and validity, multiple methods are more difficult to organize, coordinate, and carry to a conclusion than single methods. Some of these difficulties may be overcome by the use of computer databases. Multiple methods could be useful in studying HCDs such as stuttering, for which there are a variety of behavioral and neurophysiological manifestations.

References

Statistical Power Analysis:

Cohen, J. (1988). *Statistical power analysis for the behavioral sciences* (2nd ed.). Hillsdale, NJ: Erlbaum.

Kroll, R. M., & Chase, L. J. (1975). Communication disorders: A power-analytic assessment of recent research. *Journal of Communication Disorders, 8,* 237–247.

Meta-analysis:

Bat-Chava, Y. (1993). Antecedents of self-esteem in deaf people: A meta-analytic review. *Rehabilitation Psychology, 38,* 221–234.

Cooper, H., & Hedges, L. V. (Eds.). (1994). *The handbook of research synthesis.* New York: Russell Sage Foundation.

Eysenck, H. J. (1995). Meta-analysis squared—Does it make sense? *American Psychologist, 50,* 110–111.

Hattie, J. A., & Hansford, B. C. (1984). Meta-analysis: A reflection on problems. *Australian Journal of Psychology, 36,* 239–254.

Hunter, J. E., & Schmidt, F. L. (1990). *Methods of meta-analysis.* Newbury Park, CA: Sage.

Robey, R. (1994). The efficacy of treatment for aphasic persons: A meta-analysis. *Brain and Language, 47,* 582–608.

Rosenthal, R. (1991). *Meta-analytic procedures for social research* (rev. ed.). Newbury Park, CA: Sage.

Schmidt, F. L. (1992). What do data really mean? *American Psychologist, 47,* 1173–1181.

Sohn, D. (1995). Meta-analysis as a means of discovery. *American Psychologist, 50,* 108–110.

Wachter, K. W., & Straf, M. L. (Eds.). (1990). *The future of meta-analysis.* New York: Russell Sage Foundation.

Multiple Methods:

Angus, L. E. (1992). Metaphor and the communication interaction in psychotherapy: A multimethodological approach. In S. G. Toukmanian & D. L. Rennie (Eds.), *Psychotherapy process research: Paradigmatic and narrative approaches* (pp. 187–210). Newbury Park, CA: Sage.

Campbell, D. T., & Fiske, D. W. (1959). Convergent and discriminant validity by the multitrait-multimethod matrix. *Psychological Bulletin, 56,* 81–105.

Mark, M. M., & Shotland, R. L. (Eds.). (1987). *Multiple methods in program evaluation.* San Francisco: Jossey-Bass.

Rosenwald, G. C. (1988). A theory of multiple-case research. *Journal of Personality, 56,* 239–264.

Roth, P. A. (1987). *Meaning and method in the social sciences: A case for methodological pluralism.* Ithaca, NY: Cornell University Press.

Shadish, W. R. (1986). Planned critical multiplism. *Behavioral Assessment, 8,* 75–103.

Single Subject Research Methods

Single subject research designs (also called single case research designs) are appropriate for HCD treatment research because they are intended to demonstrate that interventions cause changes in behavior. A great deal of information about single subject research methods is available, with 27 texts published up until 1986 (Kratochwill & Levin, 1992), and a number since then.

Group treatment designs demonstrate treatment effects by showing a significant difference between pre- and postintervention scores, usually as compared with the scores of a control group that receives no intervention or an alternative intervention. Single subject designs assess intervention effects for individual subjects. A number of different designs are available.

In HCD research, single subject designs can be used to evaluate methods for improving communication skills or for eliminating impairments that impede communication. For example, they may be used to teach speech, hearing, and language skills to children who are hearing impaired, to help aphasic patients recover language skills, and to reduce dysfluencies in stutterers. Researchers always begin by determining a *baseline* for the *target behavior* that is to be changed. Enough measures are taken that a confident statement can be made concerning the stability of pretreatment dependent variables such as the misarticulations of children who are hearing impaired, word-finding difficulties of aphasic patients, or dysfluencies of stutterers.

When the baseline has been established, the treatment is usually applied until the target behavior changes to the desired level. The treatment must be a procedure that can be repeatedly applied, such as word repetition, picture naming, or speech timed by a metronome. Correct responses are usually rewarded in some manner. Other situational variables are carefully controlled. A change in the target behavior after a single treatment is not sufficient proof of a causal relationship between the treatment and the target behavior. Several procedures for obtaining sufficient proof will be described here. More complete details are given in Barlow and Hersen (1984), Tawney and Gast (1984), and Krishef (1991). Single subject designs in HCD research are described in McReynolds and Kearns (1983).

SINGLE SUBJECT DESIGNS

Withdrawal and Reversal Designs (ABA, ABAB)

The most basic single subject designs are *withdrawal and reversal designs*. After several baseline (A) measures, a treatment is given until the target behavior (B) changes. Then the treatment is taken away (withdrawal design) or nontarget behaviors are reinforced (reversal design) until the target behavior returns to baseline, and the treatment (B) is usually given once more. This procedure is designed to prove that the treatment caused the change in behavior. When there is baseline, treatment, and either withdrawal or reversal, it is an ABA design. When the treatment is given again after withdrawal or reversal, it is an ABAB design, which provides more complete proof of the effectiveness of treatment. These designs can be used in HCD research only when treatment effects may be temporary or can be reversed, and may be ethically inadvisable.

Multiple Baseline Designs Across Behaviors, Conditions, and Subjects

Another way to demonstrate the effect of a treatment is the multiple baseline design. Treatment effects are first demonstrated for one dependent variable, and then for two or more additional dependent variables. The additional variables can be target behaviors, conditions, or subjects.

In the *multiple baseline design across behaviors*, three or more target behaviors (e.g., the articulation of three different phonemes) are selected. Baseline measures (A) are taken for all three behaviors. Then treatment of the first target behavior (B) is begun, while baseline measures are continued for the other two behaviors. When the treatment effect for B has reached the desired level, treatment of the second target behavior (C) is begun, while baseline measures are continued for the other behavior. Finally, when target behavior C reaches the desired level, training of a third target behavior (D) can be begun, and continued until it reaches the desired level. This design is not appropriate if there is generalization from the trained target behaviors to nontrained nontarget behaviors, that is, if training a child to articulate one speech sound results in a change in the baselines for the other speech sounds. If the baseline behaviors change only when the appropriate treatment is introduced, there is evidence of a causal relationship.

In the *multiple baseline design across conditions*, a single target behavior is trained in three or more different training conditions. For example, the treatment of nonfluencies might be carried out in a research laboratory (B), at home (C), and in a public place (D). The sequence of changes from baseline measures (A) to the three conditions follows exactly the same sequence as those in the multiple baseline design across behaviors.

In the *multiple baseline design across subjects*, a baseline (A) is established for 3 or more subjects (B, C, and D), and then the treatment of a target behavior is introduced at different times for the subjects, following the sequence described for the multiple baseline design across behaviors. The multiple baseline design across subjects is frequently used in HCD research (see, e.g., Packman, Onslow, & van Doom, 1994).

As in all single subject designs, variations are possible. For example, rather than continuing baseline measures for behaviors not yet trained, baseline measures can be taken intermittently on probe trials.

Multiple Treatment Designs

The effects of two or more different treatments can be compared with several single subject designs. In some cases the treatments are given one after the other, and in other cases the treatments are trained at the same time.

The simple ABAB design can be extended to ABABC, ABABAC, ABABCD, and so forth, where new treatments are introduced after training with the first treatment. Such designs are called *multitreatment designs*. One occasion for such a design would be when the B treatment fails to result in the desired change from baseline behavior, and a new treatment C is introduced to determine whether it will work better. The usual multitreatment design involves a preplanned comparison of methods. Baselines can be taken between each treatment (ABACAD), and a theoretically optimal sequence of different treatments can be presented, such as training in imitating speech sounds followed by training in naming the speech sounds in words represented by pictures.

The *alternating treatment design*, also called the *multiple schedules design*, presents the treatments (usually only two) in each session in counterbalanced order, or in alternating sessions. It is not necessary to take baseline measures because the treatment effects are compared, but it is advisable to take the baseline measures to demonstrate the magnitude of the effects.

The *simultaneous treatment design*, also called the concurrent schedule design, is difficult to conceptualize. In an example given by Tawney and Gast (1984), simultaneous treatment involves intervention by three different persons in each training session, with each person using a different treatment.

The difficulty with multiple treatment designs in HCD research is assessing the possible carryover effects from one treatment to another in the treatment of nonreversible behaviors. This difficulty may be overcome by using different target behaviors for each treatment, for example, treatment B for one misarticulated phoneme and treatment C for a second misarticulated phoneme.

Generalization Designs

In multiple baseline designs across behaviors and conditions, generalization from one target behavior to another or from one condition to another is undesirable, because the baselines for the untrained behaviors or conditions will change. In practical training studies, however, it is hoped that training effects will not be confined to the exact targets used in training, but *will* generalize to nontrained behaviors (e.g., a phoneme correctly articulated in a set of training words will be articulated correctly in nontrained words). There are several ways of assessing generalization to nontrained behaviors in single subject designs (Barrios & Hartmann, 1988; Kratochwill & Levin, 1992). One simple method is to probe nontrained behaviors during baseline, at intervals during training, and after training. If training is done in a laboratory setting, it is important to assess generalization, that is, carryover, to a normal conversational setting.

VISUAL ANALYSIS

The basic idea behind single subject research is that experimental conditions are so well controlled that there is a very stable baseline prior to treatment and an immediate change of considerable magnitude in the target behavior as soon treatment is introduced. Then, the further procedures involved in ABAB, multiple baseline, and multiple treatment designs confirm the treatment effects. Further proof is obtained if the effect can be replicated with equally clear results. Such results can easily be seen when presented in visual form (Parsonsons & Baer, 1992).

Problems in demonstrating proof by means of visual analysis arise when the baseline is not stable and treatment effects are not immediate and large. In such cases, single subject designs may not be appropriate for the problem. In multiple treatment designs, the effects of the different treatments may be so similar that no conclusions can be reached via visual analysis regarding their relative efficacy.

STATISTICAL ANALYSIS

It can be argued that if single subject data are sufficiently variable that statistical analysis is needed to confirm treatment effects, the single subject design is inappropriate. However, a great deal has been written concerning the statistical analysis of single subject data, and such procedures might be useful in particular cases. For example, Yoder, Warren, Kim, and Gazdag (1994) used a nonparametric test of multiple baseline results to compare transitional probabilities of communicative acts (see the section on sequential analysis in Chapter 19). Busk and Marascullo (1992) described statistical procedures that can be used in single subject research, but only to *supplement* visual analysis. Thus, visual analysis is the method of choice, but may be supplemented by statistical analyses.

META-ANALYSIS

A major difficulty in single subject research is to generalize from single cases to the population under consideration. Meta-analysis has been proposed as a way to evaluate treatment effects across subjects both within and between studies (Busk & Serlin, 1992). The main technical problem is how to obtain a measure of effect size comparable to those obtained from group studies. Busk and Serlin proposed three measures, the simplest of which is quite ingenious. Pretreatment variance is expressed in terms of the standard deviation of baseline measures, and the treatment effect is the mean of the measures taken during treatment. Effect size is the mean treatment effect divided by the standard deviation of the baseline measures. If sufficient single subject data on the same topic are available, meta-analysis may prove useful for generalizing the findings beyond single cases.

ADVANTAGES AND DISADVANTAGES

Single subject designs have some of the advantages of group designs and some of the advantages of observational and case study designs. They provide direct quantitative measures of the behaviors studied, being averaged neither across subjects in groups nor across studies. Experimental conditions are rigorously controlled to obtain information about causal relationships between independent and dependent variables. Large groups of subjects are not needed. Information is obtained for individuals rather than groups. The information may have direct practical applications.

Single subject designs have their own inherent limitations. Stable baselines may be difficult to establish. If the treatment is not immediately effective in changing the baseline behavior, it may be difficult to demonstrate causal relationships. Reversal designs cannot be used if treatment effects do not or should not reverse. Multiple baseline designs cannot be used if treatment effects generalize to nontreated behaviors. Multiple treatment designs may yield ambiguous results if treatment effects carry over and if differences between treatment effects are not clear-cut. The very rigid specification of target behaviors, treatments, and control procedures may make the treatment too artificial for direct application to clinical intervention. The treatment may change the target behaviors only in the experimental situation and not in natural communication situations. Finally, there is the problem of generalizing the results. There is no way of predicting that all subjects of the same type will show the same treatment effects. Informed guesswork is unavoidable in interpreting the results of single subject research.

CONCLUSIONS

HCD researchers have made good use of single subject designs and should keep them in mind when planning research for which it is necessary to demonstrate causal relationships. There are a variety of designs, and ingenious researchers may think of further variations. Some of the limitations of these designs may be overcome if they are used in combination with other designs. If sufficient subjects are available, a group design can be combined with a single subject design and the results presented both in the form of a visual analysis of individual data and a statistical analysis of group data (see, e.g., Perigoe, 1994).

References

Barlow, D. H., & Hersen, M. (1984). *Single case experimental designs* (2nd ed.). New York: Pergamon.

Barrios, B. A., & Hartmann, D. P. (1988). Recent developments in single subject methodology: Methods for analyzing generalization, maintenance, and multi-component treatments. In M. Hersen, R. M. Eisler, & P. M. Miller (Eds.), *Progress in behavior modification* (Vol. 22, pp. 11–47). New York: Academic Press.

Busk, P. L., & Marascul_lo, L. A. (1992). Statistical analysis in single-case research. In T. R. Kratochwill & J. R. Levin (Eds.), *Single-case research: New directions for psychology and education* (pp. 159–186). Hillsdale, NJ: Erlbaum.

Busk, P. L., & Serlin, R. C. (1992). Meta-analysis for single-case research. In T. R. Kratochwill & J. R. Levin (Eds.), *Single-case research: New directions for psychology and education* (pp. 187–212). Hillsdale, NJ: Erlbaum.

Kratochwill, T. R., & Levin, J. R. (Eds.). (1992). *Single-case research: New directions for psychology and education*. Hillsdale, NJ: Erlbaum.

Krishef, C. H. (1991). *Fundamental approaches to single subject design and analysis*. Malabar, FL: Robert E. Krieger.

McReynolds, L. J., & Kearns, K. P. (1983). *Single-subject experimental designs in communicative disorders.* Baltimore: University Park Press.

Packman, A., Onslow, M., & van Doom, J. (1994). Prolonged speech and modification of stuttering: Perceptual, acoustic, and electroglottographic data. *Journal of Speech and Hearing Research, 37,* 724–737.

Parsonsons, B. S., & Baer, D. B. (1992). The visual analysis of data, and current research into the stimuli controlling it. In T. R. Kratochwill & J. R. Levin (Eds.), *Single-case research: New directions for psychology and education* (pp. 15–40). Hillsdale, NJ: Erlbaum.

Perigoe, C. B. (1994). *Effectiveness of two phonologic speech training strategies for hearing-impaired children.* Unpublished PhD dissertation, McGill University, Montreal.

Tawney, J. W., & Gast, D. L. (1984). *Single subject research in special education.* Columbus, OH: Merrill.

Yoder, P. J., Warren, S. F., Kim, K., & Gazdag, G. E. (1994). Facilitating prelinguistic communication skills in young children with development delay. II: Systematic replication and extension. *Journal of Speech and Hearing Research, 37,* 841–851.

Qualitative
Research
Methods

The term *qualitative* is used in two different senses in HCD research. Qualitative *data* include information in categories, such as male and female, as opposed to continuous measures such as height, weight, test scores, and hearing levels. Qualitative categorical data can easily be converted to quantitative frequency counts. Then statistical analysis can be carried out, usually by nonparametric tests.

The present chapter is concerned with qualitative *methods* (Denzin & Lincoln, 1994). *Quantitative* methods, as described in Part I, involve objective, verifiable observations in carefully controlled situations that yield statements of the probability of the phenomena in question, such as treatment effects. *Qualitative* methods involve subjective observations of natural situations that are analyzed and interpreted in terms of their meaning. Most current research problems in HCDs lend themselves most easily to quantitative methods. However, qualitative methods can be usefully applied to problems concerning phenomena not easily assessed by objective observations. Such phenomena include the thoughts, feelings, values, attitudes, and communicative intentions of persons with HCDs; the reactions of family, friends, and society in general to HCDs; the ways in which HCDs are viewed in different cultures; and the everyday context of communicative interactions.

Qualitative methods have been used in anthropology, sociology, and phenomenological psychology for many years, but only in the 1980s were these methods brought to the attention of the other human sciences.

Arguments for adopting qualitative methods often take the form of attacks against the philosophy of science on which quantitative research methods are based, wherein absolute truth concerning causal relationships is sought by rigorous empirical methods like those of the physical sciences. Advocates of qualitative methods feel that the objective search for truth by highly controlled observations in artificial situations cannot capture the subtlety and richness of human experience in its natural context.

The greatest strength of qualitative methods is that they open the whole realm of human experience to researchers. Researchers who espouse quantitative methods were quick to point out that this is also the greatest weakness of qualitative methods. Uncontrolled observations and subjective interpretations by fallible, possibly biased observers do not provide the kind of information that can be generalized with specified levels of confidence from the sample studied to the population in question.

Fortunately, many quantitative and qualitative researchers are coming to adopt the criterion of practical usefulness in decisions regarding research methods, leaving philosophical arguments to others. Several qualitative methods are of potential use to HCD researchers. Before these are described, it is necessary to consider how data are gathered for qualitative analyses.

DATA COLLECTION

The data used by qualitative researchers can be gathered in a number of ways—by observing or videotaping individuals and groups in natural and structured settings; by interviews; and by texts such as narratives, diaries, autobiographies, and archival information. Qualitative researchers recommend using more than one type of qualitative data, that is, both observations and interviews. This procedure, called *triangulation*, helps to establish validity and reliability.

Observation in Natural and Structured Settings

Qualitative information may be obtained from observation in natural or structured settings (Adler & Adler, 1994). Qualitative observers do their best to set aside preconceived attitudes and adopt the perspectives of the persons being observed. Hypotheses are often generated by the observations rather than specified in advance. Videotapes are extremely helpful, because they can be reviewed during all stages of data analysis and interpreted by other researchers.

Although observations are usually considered to be uncontrolled, some control may be involved in the selection of the situation to be observed. For example, a family rather than a school setting could be selected. Further control may be exerted by structuring the situation, for example, having a child who is hearing impaired play with a child who is not.

Interviews

In quantitative research, interviews are highly structured. The hypotheses to be tested and the exact role of the interviewer are specified in advance. In qualitative research, the interview is largely unstructured apart from the choice of a topic. The role of interviewer is to make the informant feel comfortable, encourage the informant to explore relevant material, and request clarification of ambiguous statements. As in unstructured observation, the interviewer makes every attempt to enter the situation without preconceived hypotheses and to adopt the perspective of the informant (Fontana & Frey, 1994).

If the interview is open ended, it may vary from one-half hour to several hours, and there may be more than one interview. The number of people interviewed depends on the topic. The focus of the interview is on the everyday experiences of the informant. An example would be the experiences of a person who is hearing impaired in an educational setting. The interviewer is open to unexpected descriptions and tries to focus on actual situations and actions rather than the informant's interpretations and theories. The interview data may be recorded in the form of notes, audiotapes, or videotapes, depending on the topic and the researcher's aims.

Interviews may fall somewhere between highly structured and completely open ended, depending on the purpose of the research. For example, subtopics such as attitudes of family, friends, and strangers toward stuttering, may be elicited rather than letting them emerge.

Texts

Written accounts, for example, of the experience of having an HCD can provide different qualitative data because the informants have more opportunity to think about the topic and revise their opinions. The written account may be a diary, a personal history, or some other type of

written or spoken narrative. Some structure may be imposed by suggestions regarding the scope of the narrative and subtopics to be discussed
(Clandinin & Connolly, 1994).

The informant may be more free to explore the topic in question in
written accounts than in interviews, but may, as a result, be more likely
to wander from the topic, be ambiguous, and offer theories and interpretations rather than descriptions of actual experiences.

DATA ANALYSIS

Qualitative information is not analyzed statistically. The analyzers are
the researchers themselves, who proceed through a series of steps to
arrive at subjective interpretations. The steps vary somewhat as a function of the method. Four methods are briefly described here for illustrative purposes. There are other methods, and the distinction between
methods is not always clear.

Ethnographic Methods

Unstructured observations usually provide the primary information for
ethnographic analyses, which were devised for the anthropological study of
different cultures. Supplementary information in the form of interviews
or texts is also used. The data are reviewed by the researchers as many
times as necessary. As the researchers discover categories, subcategories,
and components of meaning in the observations, broad themes emerge
that describe the major outlines of the phenomena observed. Ethnographic methods are especially applicable to the study of the social and
cultural context of HCDs (Crago & Cole, 1991; Fetterman, 1989).

Phenomenological Methods

Phenomenological methods were developed for studying the essential nature
of individual experiences such as anger, imagination, and approval, and
as such would be appropriate for studying individuals' feelings about their
HCDs. Interviews or texts rather than observations provide the necessary
data. There are several procedures for data analysis, which consist of steps
quite similar to those of ethnographic data analysis. Researchers read
through informants' statements to get a sense of the whole. Then the
statements are classified into categories. The next step is to reduce and

transform the informants' statements into more precise descriptive terms. Finally, the descriptive units are synthesized into a single general structural description of the experience under study (Polkinghorne, 1989).

Grounded Theory

Grounded theory is a method of analyzing qualitative data derived from ethnographic and phenomenological methods, with the explicit aim of building theories from qualitative data (Strauss & Corbin, 1994). Data analysis begins once more with developing basic descriptive categories, followed by creative thinking to relate the categories to each other and integrate them in a way that leads to a coherent theory.

Hermeneutics

Hermeneutics is a method that was developed for interpreting theological texts and later applied to literary texts. More recently it has been applied to the understanding of meaning systems in general (Packer & Addison, 1989). The purpose of hermeneutic analysis is not to understand a specific experience in itself, but to determine how meaning systems overlap and are interconnected. A given process such as anxiety is examined by the use of different sources of qualitative information, which could include written texts or the researchers' own experiences, to achieve a multidimensional understanding of the process. The next stage is to describe how the process is similar to and different from other processes. A final stage of "intuitive understanding" can be represented as overlapping circles. This creates new questions, and a *hermeneutic circle* of continually emerging information and interpretation results in an ever-broadening understanding of the experience under investigation. Hermeneutics could be useful in studying the interconnections of experiences and contexts involved in HCDs.

USE OF COMPUTERS

There has been considerable attention to the use of computers in qualitative research (Fielding & Lee, 1993; Richards & Richards, 1994). They are of obvious use in the first stage of data analysis, when data are organized into categories. Data in written form are easily stored, retrieved, and compared in separate windows with general-purpose word processors. After categories are established, they can be coded for later retrieval. With sophisticated word processors, videotaped and audiotaped data can be managed in the same manner. Search programs can be used to search for strings of text, and database management systems can be used to classify categorized data.

Special purpose qualitative analysis software has been developed for coding and retrieval of categories and then proceeding to the next stage of analysis. The systems for further analysis are similar to knowledge-based systems in artificial intelligence, and are designated as rule-based, logic-based, index-based, and conceptual network systems (Richards & Richards, 1994). Categories and subcategories of data can be organized in hierarchical tree structures or box-and-arrow diagrams. As computer systems and artificial intelligence methods develop further, more complex programs for analyzing qualitative data will become available.

There is some danger that the purposes of qualitative research will be subverted by computer data analysis systems, as opposed to researchers who keep going over the richly detailed data until intuitive understanding is reached. On the other hand, the sophisticated data analysis systems may provide new insights, and researchers with combined interests in computers, artificial intelligence, and direct access to natural phenomena may be attracted to qualitative research.

QUALITATIVE RESEARCH IN HCD

There has been considerable interest in the use of qualitative methods in HCD research (Crago & Cole, 1991; Eastwood, 1988; Kovarsky & Crago, 1990–91; Kovarsky, Maxwell, & Damico, 1993; Westby & Erickson, 1992), and a newsletter, *Ethnotes,* was established in 1990 at the University of Illinois for professionals interested in studying communication disorders from an ethnographic perspective.

Two examples will indicate the manner in which qualitative methods are used in HCD research. Pickering (1984) studied interpersonal communication in supervisory conferences. Audiotaped supervisory conferences were analyzed according to four a priori concepts and three concepts that emerged during data analysis. To verify the findings (triangulation), supervisors wrote about interpersonal communication following each conference, and the initial analysis was repeated by two associates of the author. It was found that discussions about clients in supervisory conferences did include a focus on interpersonal relationships between students and clients. Foster, Barefoot, and DeCaro (1989) studied the meaning of communication to a group of deaf college students. Ethnographic methods were used to interview the students. Analysis of the interviews organized the students' comments into four dimensions of communication, including language modality, affective, situational, and sociopolitical. These dimensions were then used to develop a multidimensional perspective on communication for use in communication training programs for deaf people.

ADVANTAGES AND DISADVANTAGES

Qualitative methods are said to overcome the limitations of quantitative methods in providing direct access to the subtlety, complexity, and richness of human experience. In this sense, qualitative methods have more ecological validity than quantitative methods. However, they require subjective decisions and reasoning that may prove difficult to verify, replicate, and generalize. The disadvantages of quantitative and qualitative methods can be overcome, at least to some extent, by using both. For example, the findings of qualitative research may suggest quantitative research that will provide further information regarding the generality of the phenomena.

CONCLUSIONS

HCD researchers should be aware of the potential usefulness of qualitative methods. They may become more applicable to HCD research as more is learned about the complexities of human experience.

References

Adler, P. A., & Adler, P. (1994). Observational techniques. In N. K. Denzin & Y. S. Lincoln (Eds.), Handbook of qualitative research (pp. 377–392). Thousand Oaks, CA: Sage.

Clandinin, D. J., & Connolly, F. M. (1994). Personal experience methods. In D. K. Denzin & Y. S. Lincoln (Eds.), Handbook of qualitative research (pp. 413–427). Thousand Oaks, CA: Sage.

Crago, M. B., & Cole, E. (1991). Using ethnography to bring children's communicative and cultural worlds into focus. In T. M. Gallagher (Ed.), *Pragmatics of language* (pp. 99–131). San Diego: Singular.

Denzin, N. K., & Lincoln, Y. S. (Eds.). (1994). *Handbook of qualitative research.* Thousand Oaks, CA: Sage.

Eastwood, J. (1988). Qualitative research: An additional research methodology for speech pathology? *British Journal of Disorders of Communication, 23,* 171–184.

Fetterman, D. M. (1989). *Ethnography: Step by step.* Newbury Park, CA: Sage.

Fielding, N. G., & Lee, R. M. (Eds.). (1991). *Using computers in qualitative research.* London: Sage.

Fontana, A., & Frey, J. H. (1994). Interviewing: The art of science. In N. K. Denzin & Y. S. Lincoln (Eds.), *Handbook of qualitative research* (pp. 316–376). Thousand Oaks, CA: Sage.

Foster, S., Barefoot, S. M., & DeCaro, P. M. (1989). The meaning of communication to deaf college students: A multidimensional perspective. *Journal of Speech and Hearing Disorders, 54,* 558–569.

Kovarsky, D., & Crago, M. (1990–91). Toward the ethnography of communication disorders. *National Student Speech Language Hearing Association Journal, 18,* 44–55.

Kovarsky, D., Maxwell, M., & Damico, S. (1993). *Language interactions in clinical and educational settings.* ASHA Monographs No. 30. Rockville, MD: American Speech-Language-Hearing Association.

Packer, M. J., & Addison, R. B. (Eds.). (1989). *Entering the circle: Hermeneutic investigation in psychology.* Albany: State University of New York Press.

Pickering, M. (1984). Interpersonal communication in speech–language pathology supervisory conferences: A qualitative study. *Journal of Speech and Hearing Disorders, 49,* 189–195.

Polkinghorne, D. (1989). Phenomenological research methods. In R. S. Valle & S. Halling (Eds.), *Existential–phenomenological perspectives in psychology* (pp. 41–60). New York: Plenum.

Richards, T. J., & Richards, L. (1994). Using computers in qualitative research. In N. K. Denzin & Y. S. Lincoln (Eds.), *Handbook of qualitative research* (pp. 445–462). Thousand Oaks, CA: Sage.

Strauss, A., & Corbin, J. (1994). Grounded theory methodology: An overview. In N. K. Denzin & Y. S. Lincoln (Eds.), *Handbook of qualitative research* (pp. 273–285). Thousand Oaks, CA: Sage.

Westby, C., & Erickson, J. (Eds.). (1992). Changing paradigms in language-learning disabilities: The role of ethnography. *Topics in Language Disorders, 12* (3).

Path Analysis, Maximum Likelihood Estimation, Loglinear Analysis, and Sequential Analysis

Several other methods that could prove useful for HCD researchers are discussed in this chapter. The methods are interrelated. For example, path analysis involves maximum likelihood estimation and sequential analysis can involve loglinear analysis. Most of the methods explicitly involve tests of *goodness-of-fit* between predicted and observed events, as well as inferences about causal relationships. These methods could, therefore, be useful for studying important problems. Methods other than those described in this book could also be useful for HCD research. New research methods are described in journals concerned with methodology such as the *Psychological Bulletin*, *Psychological Methods* (a new journal of the American Psychological Association), and *Psychometrika*.

PATH ANALYSIS

An important goal of HCD research is to determine the causes of disorders. Some inferences concerning causality can be made by the use of standard group designs, but it is usually difficult to satisfy all of the criteria for causality (see Chapter 7). Simple correlations do not permit inferences concerning causality. However, correlational methods of causal analysis have been developed and are used in many areas of human science.

Correlational methods for causal analysis are described by a somewhat confusing array of terms, including *causal modeling, path analysis, linear structural analysis*, and *latent variable structural analysis*. They all involve special applications of multivariate correlational procedures (Dillon & Goldstein, 1984; Kline, 1991). For simplicity, the term *path analysis* will be used here to describe all of these methods, although some writers prefer the more general term *latent variable structural analysis*. Fortunately, the basic concepts are not too difficult, and the calculations, although complex, can be done by computer programs.

The LISREL model (Joreskog & Sorbom, 1989) is a general, complex causal model used for path analysis. The model hypothesizes *causal paths* in terms of connections between causes and effects. The causes are *exogenous* independent variables, and the effects are *endogenous* dependent variables. For example, the exogenous variables in a causal model might be verbal intelligence and motivation, and the endogenous variables might be job performance and job satisfaction. These variables are called *latent* variables, because they are unobservable and cannot, therefore, be directly measured. The latent variables are estimated on the basis of observable and measurable *manifest* variables, such as standardized intelligence tests. To increase the reliability and validity of estimates of latent variables, multiple measures of manifest variables are often used.

The hypothesized relationships between manifest and latent exogenous and endogenous variables constitute the causal models tested by latent structural analysis. A simple model would have the components shown in Table 19–1. The causal model specifies the relationships between the manifest and latent exogenous and endogenous variables.

Path analysis by use of the LISREL computer program (Joreskog & Sorbom, 1989) involves three steps. First, the observed covariance matrix is calculated. Then this covariance matrix is compared with a *reproduced* covariance matrix predicted by the model. Finally, the *goodness-of-fit* of the observed and predicted covariance matrices is tested by a *maximum likelihood estimation* procedure (Dillon & Goldstein, 1984; Kline, 1991).

Path Analysis in HCD Research

Duffy, Watt, and Duffy (1994) used path analysis to test five different causal theories of pantomime deficits in aphasia. The theories involved intellectual loss, asymbolia, limb apraxia, and visual deficit as possible

TABLE 19–1. Components of a Latent Variable Structural Model
Used for Path Analysis

EXOGENOUS VARIABLES		ENDOGENOUS VARIABLES	
MANIFEST	LATENT	LATENT	MANIFEST
Measure 1	Intelligence	Job performance	Measure 1
Measure 2			Measure 2
Measure 1	Motivation	Job satisfaction	Measure 1
Measure 2			Measure 2

causes (exogenous variables), and pantomime expression deficit and pantomime recognition deficit as possible effects (endogenous variables). Their analysis was done by a LISREL model for directly observed (manifest) variables rather than unobservable (latent) variables. There was one measure for each of the exogenous and endogenous variables. The model for which observed and reproduced covariance matrices were most similar, and goodness-of-fit of the model was highest, as indicated by maximum likelihood estimation, hypothesized that pantomime expression deficits were jointly caused by limb apraxia and asymbolia, and pantomime recognition deficits were jointly caused by asymbolia and visual deficits.

Advantages and Disadvantages

Causal analyses of correlational data offer a great opportunity for gaining insight into the nature of HCDs. Like all other methods, path analysis must be used with great caution. The interpretation of findings depends on the reliability and validity of the measures of manifest variables and on the characteristics of the subjects. Duffy, Watt, and Duffy (1994) pointed out that different results might have been obtained with different populations of aphasics and different measures of the variables used in their analyses. The measures of asymbolia and intellectual deficit were particularly questionable. Another problem relates to the determination of the "best" theoretical model in terms of goodness-of-fit. There is no significance test, and better fits might be obtained with theoretical models that were not included in the analyses. However, the interesting study by Duffy, Watt, and Duffy illustrates the potential usefulness of path analysis for HCD research.

MAXIMUM LIKELIHOOD ESTIMATION

Maximum likelihood estimation is used not only in path analysis but also in a number of other procedures in which experimental data are fitted to theoretical models. It is an *iterative* procedure that systematically searches over different possible values of the population under study, selecting estimates of the values that have the maximum likelihood of fitting the observed values of the variables. There are a number of different statistical techniques for maximum likelihood estimates. Computer programs are needed to carry out the complex and lengthy calculations (Eliason, 1993).

Applications of maximum likelihood estimation include the extraction of factors to confirm a model of the structure of the intellect (Chen & Michael, 1993), the estimation of genetic and environmental influences on twins (Cherny, DeFries, & Fulker, 1992), estimation of the sensitivity and specificity of four diagnostic techniques used in psychiatry (Streiner & Miller, 1990), and in estimations of expertise and experience with microcomputers (DeSarbo, Howard, & Jedidi, 1991).

Bates and her colleagues have made extensive use of maximum likelihood estimation in HCD research (Bates & Appelbaum, 1994; Bates, McDonald, MacWhinney, & Appelbaum, 1991). In one study, they formulated models of sentence comprehension to predict differences among English, German, and Italian speakers. Then they used a maximum likelihood estimation procedure to demonstrate the goodness-of-fit of the theoretical models to data collected for normal and aphasic subjects in each language group. These results agreed with results obtained by analyses of variance. Maximum likelihood estimation also demonstrated goodness-of-fit of the theoretical models to the data for individuals within each group. For both the group and individual analyses, the predictions were not as good for the subjects with aphasia as for the normal subjects.

Advantages and Disadvantages

In the study reported by Bates et al. (1991), a procedure that fits experimental data to theoretical models was used in conjunction with a standard research design. This is a clever strategy for balancing the strengths and weaknesses of each method. Maximum likelihood estimation gives more detailed theoretical information, but does not provide information about statistical significance. In addition, maximum likelihood estimation can be used for estimating goodness-of-fit for individual subjects. As with all other quantitative procedures, the findings obtained with maximum likelihood estimation are limited by the reliability and validity of the experimental measures and the samples of subjects studied.

LOGLINEAR ANALYSIS

Parametric statistical tests use data measured along continuous scales. Data organized into categories are not continuous, but must be entered into tables that show the frequency of occurrence of events in the various categories. A nonparametric test for data in frequency tables is the chi-square test, which can be used for data in two-dimensional frequency tables (see Chapter 11). The calculations and the interpretation of chi-square tests are very simple.

When categorical data are entered into frequency tables with three or more dimensions, the procedures for analysis and interpretation are much more complex. A procedure called *loglinear analysis* is commonly used for analyzing multidimensional frequency data (Dillon & Goldstein, 1984; Tabachnick & Fidell, 1989). Computer programs are available to make the researchers' task easier (Bakeman & Robinson, 1994). The analysis begins by carrying out tests of the goodness-of-fit between observed and expected cell frequencies for the maximum number of dimensions. If no significant relationships are found, the tests are repeated for lower dimensional frequency tables until significant relationships are found.

A hypothetical example will indicate how this technique might be usefully applied in HCD research. In the study by Gertner, Rice, and Hadley (1994) described in connection with the sequence of research events in Chapter 3, three groups of preschool children were compared in terms of their popularity with classmates. If the data had been expressed in categories, the relation between group membership and popularity could have been easily assessed by a two-dimensional chi-square test, with two categories (popular and unpopular) for one dimension and three categories (normal development, specific language impairment, and children with English as a second language) for the other dimension.

To extend the two-dimensional frequency table for loglinear analysis, two other dimensions could be added—age (3 and 4) and social skills training (trained and untrained). This would result in a four-dimensional frequency table, as shown in Table 19–2. The original two-dimensional table with six cells has been increased to three dimensions involving two six-cell tables by adding the variable of social skills training, and further increased to four dimensions involving four six-cell tables by adding the variable of age.

Loglinear analysis would begin by comparing the observed and expected frequencies for the four-dimensional table. A significant result could occur here if social skills training affected popularity for the 4-year-olds but not the 3-year-olds, and if popularity varied among the three groups of preschool children (the original finding of Gertner, Rice, & Hadley, 1994). If, however, social skills training affected the popularity of 3- and 4-year-olds in the same way, the four-dimensional analysis would be non-significant, and the data would be collapsed into three-dimensional tables.

If social skills training had no effect, the three-dimensional analysis would also be nonsignificant, and the data would be collapsed into the original two-dimensional tables. If the results of this study were the same as those of Gertner, Rice, and Hadley (1994), the two-dimensional log-linear analysis (or a chi-square analysis) might show a significant relationship between popularity and group membership.

TABLE 19–2. 2 × 3 × 2 × 2 Frequency Table for a Study of Popularity in Preschool Children

		Trained Popular	Trained Unpopular	Untrained Popular	Untrained Unpopular
Age 3	Normal development				
	Specific language impairment				
	English second language				
Age 4	Normal development				
	Specific language impairment				
	English second language				

Advantages and Disadvantages

Loglinear analysis has the advantage of all nonparametric tests. Because the data are frequencies, there are no assumptions regarding the distributions of the variables. It has an additional advantage of assessing interactions between variables. For the example in Table 19–2, loglinear analysis assessed the interactive effects of age, social skills training, and group memberships on popularity.

Although potentially very useful, loglinear analysis has a number of disadvantages. Like all nonparametric tests, it is not as powerful as parametric tests involving continuous measures. If the results of the loglinear analysis of the highest dimension frequency table are nonsignificant, it cannot be concluded that there is no effect, because the measures may not have been sufficiently sensitive to show an effect. Multidimensional analyses may require too many subjects. A very rough estimate would be an average of 10 subjects per cell. With this criterion, a minimum of 240 subjects would be required for the hypothetical study in Table 19–2.

SEQUENTIAL ANALYSIS

Communicative interactions such as conversations between two persons have been studied as *sequential dyadic interactions*. The term *serial dependence* has been used to describe the effects that each member of the dyad has on the other's behavior (Iacobucci & Wasserman, 1988). If the measures of behavior are continuous, a parametric technique called *time-series analysis* is used; and if the measures of behavior are categorical, nonparametric techniques called *sequential analysis* are used. Both methods are described in Bakeman and Gottman (1986) and Gottman and Roy (1990). Sequential analysis is described here.

Like the other methods described in this chapter, the basic idea behind sequential analysis is fairly simple, but the exact manner in which the analyses are carried out can involve difficult decisions and complex computations, for which computer programs are available (Gottman & Roy, 1990). The first step in sequential analysis is to decide on the exact behaviors that are to be studied. Researchers have to begin with a specific question regarding dyadic interactions, specify the behaviors manifested in the interactions, and develop a coding scheme that can enable observers to reliably identify the behaviors during communicative interactions.

After the interactions have been observed, there are two steps of data analysis. The first step, unique to sequential analysis, involves the calculation of *transitional probabilities*. The simplest form of transitional probability is based on the frequency with which a particular event B—the target event—follows an event A. There can be much more complex transitional probabilities involving more than two events and two participants, as well as events that do not immediately follow one another.

In sequential analysis, transitional probabilities are treated as descriptive statistics. Inferential statistics must be used to determine the statistical significance of the observed relationships between interactive events. A number of different statistical techniques have been used, ranging from simple standardized scores to complex procedures such as maximum likelihood estimation of loglinear models (Bakeman & Gottman, 1986; Gottman & Roy, 1990; Iacobucci & Wasserman, 1988). The more complex statistics are used for transitional probabilities of multiple events associated with multiple dyadic interactions.

The basic question asked in sequential analysis is, however, straightforward and important. How much are particular behaviors of one member of the dyad (or triad, etc.) likely to affect the behaviors of the other member? In studies of the interactions of married couples, for example, it was found that the wife's behavior was better predicted from the husband's behavior than vice versa. This was called a "dominance effect" (surely not universal), and as such illustrates that sequential analysis is a form of causal analysis (Iacobucci & Wasserman, 1988).

Sequential Analysis in HCD Research

Yoder, Warren, Kim, and Gazdag (1994) used sequential analysis in studying the prelinguistic communicative skills of 4 children with developmental delay. They used a single subject design (multiple baseline across subjects) to facilitate prelinguistic intentional requests. The intervention was aimed at teaching the children to make prelinguistic requests such as looking at a cup and then looking at the researcher. After these behaviors had been established over a number of sessions, the researchers observed the children's communicative interactions with their mother and with a teacher, both of whom were unaware of the training procedures and the purpose of the study.

The increase in prelinguistic requests generalized from the training sessions to the sessions with mothers and teachers. The transitional probability that was studied was whether behavior A—the child's intentional request—was predictive of (that is, caused an increase in) behavior B— the *linguistic mapping of child communication* by the mother and teacher. Linguistic mapping occurred, for example, if the child looked at the cup and then at the adult, and then the adult linguistically mapped the child's behavior by saying, "You want the cup."

Transitional probabilities were determined from the proportion of times the child's intentional acts were followed by linguistic mapping by the adult. As a control, transitional probabilities were also determined from the proportion of times "preintentional acts" (in which, for example, the child looked at either the cup or the adult, but not both) were followed by linguistic mapping by the adult.

The transitional probabilities for linguistic mapping after intentional acts were larger than those after preintentional acts for all the child–adult dyads. The difference in transitional probabilities for this very small sample, as determined by a one-tailed Wilcoxon nonparametric test (Chapter 11), was significant at the .05 level. Thus, Yoder et al. (1994) demonstrated that after prelinguistic intentional requesting had been increased by special training, the change in the child's behavior led to a change in the mother's and teacher's behavior. The researchers cited previous research suggesting that the increase in linguistic mapping of child communication would in time be likely to facilitate vocabulary development.

Advantages and Disadvantages

Sequential analysis can be very useful for studying communicative inter-actions in terms of transitional probabilities. However, the interactive behaviors to be studied must be precisely defined on the basis of prior knowledge, the reliability of observations must be ensured, and the methods of determining statistical significance may be very complex.

Conclusions

The example of HCD research involving sequential analysis provides a very fitting conclusion to the consideration of research methods. Yoder and his colleagues are superb research strategists. The problem of facili-tating communicative development in children with developmental delay is very important. Their decisions regarding the specific purpose of the research and their interpretation of the results required extensive knowledge of theories and research concerning language development. Their purpose was accomplished through a judicious blend of single subject research methods, observational methods, sequential analysis, and nonparametric statistical analysis. Their interpretation was cautious and self-critical.

References

Path Analysis:

Dillon, W. R., & Goldstein, M. (1984). *Multivariate analysis*. New York: Wiley.

Duffy, R. J., Watt, J. H., & Duffy, J. R. (1994). Testing causal theories of pantomimic deficits in aphasia using path analysis. *Aphasiology, 8*, 361–379.

Joreskog, K., & Sorbom, D. (1989). *LISREL 7 user's reference guide*. Mooresville, IN: Scientific Software.

Kline, R. B. (1991). Latent variable path analysis in clinical psychology: A beginner's tour guide. *Journal of Clinical Psychology, 47*, 471–484.

Maximum Likelihood Estimation:

Bates, E., & Appelbaum, M. (1994). Methods of studying small samples. In S. H. Broman & J. Grafman (Eds.), *Atypical cognitive deficits in developmental disorders* (pp. 245–280). Hillsdale, NJ: Erlbaum.

Bates, E., McDonald, J., MacWhinney, B., & Appelbaum, M. (1991). A maximum likelihood procedure for the analysis of group and individual data in aphasia research. *Brain and Language, 40*, 231–265.

Chen, S. A., & Michael, W. B. (1993). First order and higher-order factors of creative social intelligence within Guilford's structure-of-intellect model: A reanalysis of a Guilford data base. *Educational and Psychological Measurement, 53*, 619–641.

Cherny, S. S., DeFries, J. C., & Fulker, D. W. (1992). Multiple regression analysis of twin data: A model-fitting approach. *Behavior Genetics, 22*, 489–497.

DeSarbo, W. S., Howard, D. J., & Jedidi, K. (1991). MULTICLUS: A new method for simultaneously performing multidimensional scaling and cluster analysis. *Psychometrika, 56*, 121–136.

Eliason, S. R. (1993). *Maximum likelihood estimation: Logic and practice*. Newbury Park, CA: Sage.

Streiner, D. L., & Miller, H. R. (1990). Maximum likelihood estimates of the accuracy of four diagnostic instruments. *Educational and Psychological Measurement, 50*, 653–662.

Loglinear Analysis:

Bakeman, R., & Robinson, B. F. (1994). *Understanding log-linear analysis with ILOG*. Hillsdale, NJ: Erlbaum.

Dillon, W. R., & Goldstein, M. (1984). *Multivariate analysis*. New York: Wiley.

Tabachnick, B. G., & Fidell, L. S. (1989). *Using multivariate statistics* (2nd ed.). New York: HarperCollins.

Sequential Analysis:

Bakeman, R., & Gottman, J. M. (1986). *Observing interaction: An introduction to sequential analysis*. New York: Cambridge University Press.

Gottman, J. M., & Roy, A. K. (1990). *Sequential analysis: A guide for behavioral researchers*. New York: Cambridge University Press.

Iacobucci, D., & Wasserman, S. (1988). A general framework for the statistical analysis of sequential dyadic interaction data. *Psychological Bulletin, 103,* 379–390.

Yoder, P. J., Warren, S. F., Kim, K., & Gazdag, G. E. (1994). Facilitating prelinguistic communication skills in young children with developmental delay. II: Systematic replication and extension. *Journal of Speech and Hearing Research, 37,* 841–851.

PART III

Present and Future
Research Strategies

Research Strategies

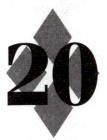

H CD research does not consist of simply carrying out a prescribed set of activities with a fixed set of research tools. Modifications and compromises are always needed to accommodate the practical problems of HCD research. The purpose, design, procedure, and method of analysis have to be adjusted and readjusted until all fit together into a study that will provide the desired information about the problem. There are many different kinds of HCD research problems. An approach that is suitable for one problem will not be appropriate for another. The flexible planning required for HCD research is better described as strategy than method.

Researchers must be concerned with all aspects of the search for knowledge, from the evaluation of the problem to the smallest details of selecting and instructing subjects and recording their responses. These activities require strategies that go beyond the specific research events discussed in previous chapters. In the beginning stages of learning to do research, there is a natural tendency to become preoccupied with the unfamiliar technicalities of particular research designs, procedures, and data analysis. To carry out effective HCD research, however, it is necessary to adopt a broad perspective concerning choices among alternatives at each stage of research. Designs, procedures, and methods of analysis are just tools, not the sum and substance of research.

How can HCD researchers learn research strategies? It is not possible for researchers to learn all there is to know about each type of design, procedure, and analysis. In all aspects of HCD research, there has to be a balance of rigor and expedience. Researchers need to become familiar with the available alternatives without becoming an expert in every method. In the planning of each stage of research, it is helpful to know enough about the various methods to consider each alternative before reaching a decision. Then whatever additional information is required can be obtained by referring to specialized sources of information. Familiarity with each research event is necessary. For example, researchers who do not understand methods of data analysis can make serious mistakes in both designing and interpreting research. Researchers who are not familiar with strategies, methods, and techniques relevant to the problem place themselves at a disadvantage. The same is true for researchers who have learned only one research approach and apply it to all problems.

Thoughtfulness is an essential component of HCD research strategy. Before reaching decisions about each research event and agreeing on the final integrated plan, researchers need to do as much careful, constructive thinking as possible. Equal thoughtfulness is required for interpreting the findings. The most important contribution to knowledge may be the realization of what is *not* known.

An essential aspect of research strategy is continuing sensitivity to the degree of uncertainty involved in research. Researchers can have no prior assurance that they will achieve new knowledge. When planning research, however, they should make the best possible use of what is already known about the phenomena under investigation. When previous knowledge has decreased uncertainty, specific predictions may be possible. This would permit planned comparisons, thereby increasing the power of the research. When there is less previous knowledge and more uncertainty, researchers may sacrifice analytic power in order to assess a wider range of possible effects.

In seeking the most appropriate approach to a particular problem, researchers face the prospect that a method with acceptable internal validity will not have external validity, or vice versa. In such cases, the researchers could decide to use more than one approach. When alternative approaches are used, one approach may have more internal validity and the other more external validity. A common strategy in HCD research is to obtain both descriptive information and statistically analyzed information. Statistical analyses are interpreted to arrive at definite conclusions, and the descriptive information provides suggestions for further research. Descriptive information can include detailed quantitative data that are not statistically analyzed, as well as subjective observations of the researchers and introspective reports of the subjects.

A similar strategy is to approach a particular problem from different perspectives. An example would be the problem of how to help persons with acquired sensorineural hearing loss, which can be approached from at least two different perspectives. Quantitatively oriented researchers might obtain information about the benefits of speechreading training by a series of studies that systematically vary age, gender, education, amount of hearing loss, type of training, duration of training, and other relevant variables. Qualitatively oriented researchers might instead begin by interviewing persons with acquired hearing loss, their families, their friends, and their fellow employees to assess the effects of hearing loss. They would obtain information about situational variables such as family support and the communicative demands of different settings, and personal variables such as motivation, success in self-management of problems, and risk taking in communication. Both types of approach should provide more useful knowledge about the important problem of improving the communication of persons with hearing loss.

STRATEGIES USED FOR SPECIFIC RESEARCH EVENTS

In addition to the overall strategies discussed above, it is helpful to approach each research event as a strategist.

Problem

The choice of a problem involves knowledge about research, theory, and practice related to the problem, plus thoughtful insight into the aspects of the problem most worth investigating. To have the required depth of information about particular problems, the best strategy for most researchers is to avoid studying too many different types of problems at the same time. As described in Chapter 2, there is a wide range of HCD research problems that require quite different approaches. Researchers who divide their efforts among too many different problems may tend to approach each problem in too superficial a manner.

The choice of problem will also be influenced by the researchers' general preferences regarding the type of phenomena studied. Dimensions of preference regarding different subject matter would include peripheral–central, receptive–expressive, physiological–behavioral, and assessment–intervention.

Purpose

Once a problem has been selected, research strategies play a crucial part in decisions concerning the specific purpose. The researchers must evaluate both the current state of knowledge about the problem and the available designs and procedures before deciding on the purpose. They may choose to pursue a small or a large gap in knowledge. The statement of purpose determines whether there will be carefully preplanned comparisons or open-ended searches.

Design

In the selection of research designs, the basic strategy is to be thoughtful and well informed. Researchers should not impulsively select what seems to be the one obvious best design. There is rarely a perfect design.

A series of decisions must be made in choosing the research design. The first is the general approach, which can range from quantitative to qualitative. The choice of approach is determined in part by the attitudes of the researchers. Those who prefer to be cautious, orderly, and analytic may choose a quantitative approach, whereas those who take a more holistic view may choose qualitative approaches. Among the orderly and analytic, those who wish to arrive at general conclusions about populations may choose standard group designs, and those who wish to draw rigorous conclusions about individuals may choose single subject designs. Eclectic strategists may use more than one approach.

Whatever the design, it must not be viewed as the best or the only possible approach. Dogmatic, rigid attempts to make a particular approach fit all problems will not advance knowledge as much as more flexible approaches to research design. The choice of design should be dictated by the problem and the purpose as well as the researchers' preferences.

When a particular design has been chosen, the researcher should keep in mind its advantages and disadvantages. Standard group designs that permit inferences about cause and effect may not be feasible. The designs that can be used may provide information only about relationships between the variables studied. Conclusions will usually be reached about average group performance rather than individual performance, and measures of variables may be crude and have doubtful reliability and validity. Researchers who use single subject designs should keep in mind the difficulties of generalizing from individual performance to populations and from rigidly controlled experimental operations to real-life situations. Those who use observational approaches and qualitative methods should keep in mind the difficulty of drawing general conclusions from uncontrolled observations and achieving agreement with other researchers concerning subjective observations. Whatever design is selected, the best strategy for researchers is to adopt a suitably cautious attitude.

Procedures

Strategies for selecting procedures involve balancing the need for valid and reliable procedures against the availability of subjects, tasks, equipment, facilities, and research personnel. Hasty choices dictated by practical expedience may greatly limit the interpretability of findings. Excessive concern about reliability and validity may delay or prevent the research. When the choice between these extremes is too difficult, methodological research might be needed to demonstrate the validity and reliability of procedures that meet practical needs.

Data Analysis

There is no perfect data analysis technique. As is the case for research designs, each technique has its advantages and disadvantages. Researchers must be flexible, ingenious, and well informed in selecting methods of data analysis. When statistical analyses are involved, the researchers can get supplementary information about the findings from descriptive statistics. The examination of group distributions is especially helpful for interpreting significant and nonsignificant differences, and individual results provide useful indications of the representativeness of group findings. When data are observational, researchers should not hesitate to quantify information that might be helpful in interpreting the special types of analysis required by qualitative methods.

When statistical analyses are used, the researchers have to make final decisions regarding statistical analysis at the time the research is designed. Planned comparisons should be used wherever possible, and designs that require accepting the null hypothesis should be avoided. Researchers should know the standards for statistical analyses of the professional journals to which research reports will be submitted, and make certain that the data analyses meet these standards.

Interpretation

The essential strategy for interpretation is to accomplish an orderly set of goals. Researchers should refer the findings to the stated purpose and to previous research; remain aware of the limitations imposed by the design, procedure, and data analysis; offer cautious recommendations regarding practical applications; make creative suggestions for further research; and arrive at appropriate conclusions concerning the contribution to knowledge. Specific strategies are to thoughtfully and correctly interpret interactions; be cautious about statements concerning causal relationships, correlations, and acceptance of the null hypothesis; evaluate the adequacy of relevant controls; and reach appropriate conclusions concerning the generality of findings. The findings should be interpreted in such a way that other researchers have the necessary information and are encouraged to proceed further.

THE IMPORTANCE OF SELF-CRITICISM

Proponents of a particular research method often support their arguments by criticizing other methods. Advocates of single subject designs, meta-analysis, and qualitative research criticize traditional research methods, each from a different perspective. This may imply that they consider their method the perfect method. However, responsible methodologists always point out the limitations of the methods that they advocate. Researchers should be sensitive to the limitations imposed by their strategic decisions at each stage of research. Otherwise, their research may be misleading rather than informative in the quest for a better understanding of HCDs. This self-critical approach has been used for each of the methods discussed in this book.

THE NEED FOR MULTIPLE PERSPECTIVES

The knowledge obtained by research is provisional because it is unavoidably influenced by the theories, designs, procedures, and analyses used in research, as well as the values and expectations of the researchers. To overcome the limitations of a single perspective, multiple approaches to research have been strongly recommended for both quantitative and qualitative research, as discussed in Chapters 16 and 18. Multiple perspectives converge on the essential nature of the phenomena under consideration, increasing the likelihood of useful knowledge (Polkinghorne, 1983).

References

Polkinghorne, D. (1983). *Methodology for the human sciences*. Albany: State University of New York Press.

The Future

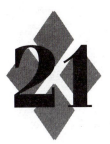

HCD research takes place in the context of changing knowledge, theories, research methods, technologies, professional practices, and cultures. Present research strategies may no longer be appropriate 10 years from now. Researchers must keep pace with new developments and be prepared to adjust their strategies.

NEW KNOWLEDGE

Generally accepted knowledge about HCDs accumulates slowly, mostly in relation to peripheral speech and hearing disorders. Knowledge about language disorders has remained provisional. However, recent advances in knowledge about language (Jackendoff, 1992; Pinker, 1994), and about genetics (Ludlow & Cooper, 1983; Crago & Gopnik, 1994) and brain function (Caplan, 1987; Tallal, 1994) in relation to language disorders, suggest that multiple methods involving linguistic, genetic, and neurological information can lead to more general knowledge about HCDs. These multiple sources of knowledge are also useful for the development of new theories concerning HCDs (Locke, 1994).

NEW RESEARCH METHODS

New methods are likely to go in two directions—more sophisticated quantitative methods (see, e.g., Grimm & Yarnold, 1995) and more highly evolved qualitative methods (see, e.g., Denzin & Lincoln, 1994). New quantitative methodology will probably involve more rigorous procedures for estimating causal relationships and evaluating theoretical models. New qualitative procedures could involve improved methods for analyzing conversations, language samples, and texts.

NEW PROCEDURES

For quantitative research, new procedures could involve the development of more reliable and valid measures of speech, language, and hearing, and of attitudes toward HCDs. For qualitative research, procedures that adapt qualitative methods for HCD research could be very helpful.

NEW TECHNOLOGIES

The technologies used in HCD research will advance as computer technology advances. Important computer applications include stimulus presentation, the control of experimental tasks, data recording, and data analysis, as well as programs that make databases and research literature universally available (McWhinnie, 1995; Stoloff & Couch, 1992). There have been great advances in all these aspects of technology. Further advances can be expected.

CULTURAL EVOLUTION

During the past century, communication has played an increasingly important part in the world's cultures. Forms and functions of communication will continue to change in a computerized world beset with political, economic, social, and ecological problems. HCD researchers and practitioners are now paying much more attention to problems associated with multiculturalism, particularly as related to HCDs associated with second language learning. As communication via computer becomes universal, the distinction between spoken and written communication may change, and HCDs may be manifested in different ways. HCD research and practice will be shaped by the changing demands of the next millennium (Csikszentmihalyi, 1993).

CONCLUSIONS

Research is a commitment to explore the unknown. It provides a difficult but rewarding opportunity to extend the frontiers of knowledge about human communication disorders.

References

Caplan, D. (1987). *Neurolinguistics and linguistic aphasiology.* New York: Cambridge University Press.

Crago, M. B., & Gopnik, M. (1994). From families to phenotypes: Theoretical and clinical implications of research into the genetic basis of specific language impairment. In R. Watkins & M. Rice (Eds.), *Specific language impairment in children* (pp. 35–51). Baltimore: Brookes.

Csikszentmihalyi, M. (1993). *The evolving self: A psychology for the third millennium.* New York: HarperCollins.

Denzin, N. K., & Lincoln, Y. S. (Eds.). (1994). *Handbook of qualitative research.* Thousand Oaks, CA: Sage.

Grimm, L. G., & Yarnold, P. (Eds.). (1995). *Reading and understanding multivariate statistics.* Washington, DC: American Psychological Association.

Jackendoff, R. S. (1992). *Languages of the mind.* Cambridge, MA: MIT Press.

Locke, J. L. (1994). Gradual emergence of developmental language disorders. *Journal of Speech and Hearing Research, 37,* 608–616.

Ludlow, C., & Cooper, J. A. (Eds.). (1983). *Genetic aspects of speech and language disorders.* New York: Academic Press.

McWhinnie, B. (1995). *The CHILDES [Child Language Data Exchange] Project* (2nd ed.). Hillsdale, NJ: Erlbaum.

Pinker, S. (1994). *The language instinct.* New York: William Morrow.

Stoloff, M. L., & Couch, J. V. (Eds.). (1992). *Computer use in psychology: A directory of software* (3rd ed.). Washington, DC: American Psychological Association.

Tallal, P. (Ed.). (1994). *Neural and cognitive mechanisms underlying speech, language, and reading.* Cambridge, MA: Harvard University Press.

APPENDIX A

How to Read and Evaluate HCD Research Reports

To be accepted for publication in an HCD journal, a research report must be reviewed by two or three experts and found to meet the journal's standards regarding the quality of research and the style of presentation. The more familiar the reader is with the content and the style of research reports, the easier they are to read and to evaluate. Knowledge of the events that take place in research, as described in the preceding chapters, also helps the reader to understand the contents of research reports. This appendix describes the style of HCD research reports, shows how to extract the information about research events from them, and gives guidelines for evaluating the research.

READING THE REPORT

Research reports must be carefully read in order to evaluate the findings of the researchers. Students read research reports to help them learn about HCDs and HCD research. Practitioners read them to learn something new about HCDs, to decide whether some aspect of their practice should be changed, and to help plan clinical research. Researchers read them to find out about current research approaches and decide what needs to be done next. Many readers combine the roles of student and researcher, or practitioner and researcher. To extract the information that is needed for these various purposes, the reader must be familiar with the different parts of research reports and know how to find the different research events.

Research reports are most often published in professional journals. The leading American HCD journal is the *Journal of Speech and Hearing Research*. Most professionals read this journal and other journals in their area of specialization to keep up with new developments in HCD research.

Research is also reported in other ways. Some projects are so large in scale that a whole book or monograph is needed. The research is reviewed by experts, but the style is less standard. Research reports are also published as chapters in books devoted to a particular topic. In such cases there may not be a careful review, and the reports are often informal and incomplete. Before research reports are published, they are often distributed privately in the form of "preprints." Such reports have not yet been reviewed but are usually written in the style of journal articles. Research is also reported in unpublished theses that have been reviewed and approved by the candidate's thesis committee.

Parts of the Research Report

The research report is supposed to describe the background of the study and then state why it was done, what was done, what was found, and how the findings relate to previous knowledge. The information has to fit into the limited space available in journals and books, usually no more than 10 or 12 pages. If this cannot be done, the researcher must publish the report in monograph or book form or circulate a privately printed report.

Research reports vary in style from one journal to another and from one form of publication to another, but most include the following parts:

- Title
- Authors
- Abstract
- Introduction
- Method
- Results
- Discussion
- Acknowledgments

- References
- Address for contacting author

To get an idea of what is included in each part, readers should look through the reports in an issue of the *Journal of Speech and Hearing Research* as each part is described here.

Title

The title may indicate something about the problem, the question, the research design, and the subjects. It may be possible to decide which papers you want to look at from the table of contents of a journal or book, or from a list of journal titles in a reference source such as *Current Contents*.

Authors

The authors are those who played a major part in finding the problem, planning the study, collecting, analyzing, and interpreting the data and writing the report. The person who did the most is usually listed first, and may be the only author. Other authors may be members of a research team, or colleagues who gave special help with one or more parts. When the institutional affiliation of the authors is given, it may provide some information about the context of the research, since many departments have well-established programs of research on certain topics.

Abstract

The abstract summarizes the study in a few hundred words, with a sentence or two about the problem, question, design, subjects, method, results, and interpretation.

Introduction

The introduction begins the actual report, usually with no heading. It puts the research in context, establishes the necessity for doing it, and tells what is to be done. The authors begin by stating the problem and reviewing the most relevant theories, research, and practical implications. They usually specify the purpose and summarize the experimental plan, and may make formal predictions about the outcome. All of this is fitted into 1 to 3 pages. The review of previous research may be longer in the case of a new or complex topic, and shorter if the study directly extends previous research. Readers may have to read some of the reports of previous research referred to in the article's introduction in order to understand the present report.

Method

The Method section is supposed to give enough detail in 1 to 3 pages so that someone else could replicate the study. It is usually divided into subsections with headings such as Subjects, Materials, Procedure, and Data Analysis, but HCD researchers often modify the headings to fit their study, as one can see by looking through an issue of the *Journal of Speech and Hearing Research*.

The Subjects subsection is usually first, but sometimes the Method section begins with an unheaded paragraph that describes the experimental design or a special technique used in the study. Such introductory paragraphs should be read carefully, because the authors have considered the material important enough to describe separately.

Subjects

Almost all research reports have a Subjects section. This is especially necessary in HCD research, because the subjects are selected from special populations. The criteria for defining the HCD must be specified, and other information relevant to the study such as age, gender, intelligence level, socioeconomic status, and information about the HCD may also be given.

Materials

Following the description of subjects, there is a description of the equipment, tests, or other materials used in the study. This section has headings such as Materials, Apparatus, Instrumentation, or Tests. The amount and type of details regarding materials depend on the study. It is important to determine the exact definitions of the independent and dependent variables. There may be reference to more complete information elsewhere. There should be enough information to permit replication.

Procedure

After subjects and materials have been described, the procedure used to collect the experimental data is described. For studies involving training, the procedures used at each stage of training are described at some length. When a single set of measurements is obtained in one testing session, the description of procedure can be shorter.

Data Analysis

In reports in which the data analysis involves special techniques or is particularly complex, the analyses are described in a subsection in the Method section. Otherwise they will first be mentioned in the Results section.

Reliability

When the data are based on the judgments of observers, it is necessary to carry out special procedures to insure that the judgments are reliable. These are often described in the Method section.

Results

After the necessary information has been given about background, design, and experimental operations, the findings of the study are presented. In experiments in which the results are not particularly complex, they may be combined with the interpretation in a section called Results and Discussion. The results are described in 1 to 4 pages, and may be divided into subsections that give the results for different groups, types of measurement procedure, or types of data analysis. The most important parts of the Results are often tables and graphs that present descriptive statistics and summarize the data analyses. These may be the essence of the findings.

Discussion

The results are interpreted in 1 to 3 pages in the Discussion section. The researchers return to the questions posed in the Introduction and decide how adequately they have answered them. Some authors stop there, but most try to relate the findings to those of previous researchers, discuss the practical and theoretical implications, and end with suggestions for further research. Some reports end with a subsection entitled Summary or Conclusions that summarizes the findings and interpretation.

Acknowledgments

Help given to authors is acknowledged in a footnote or a separate section. In the *Journal of Speech and Hearing Research*, the acknowledgments follow the Discussion. In this section, the authors acknowledge financial support by governmental agencies, private foundations, or others. They thank persons who gave advice about the research, made constructive criticisms of the written report, gave technical and clerical assistance, and provided subjects and testing or training facilities.

References

Published and unpublished books, journal articles, theses, and presentations at professional conferences referred to in the body of the paper are listed alphabetically in most journals in a standard format at the end of the research report. This section is essential. It gives information that may be needed to understand the background of the research report.

Appendixes

Appendixes are sometimes inserted after the references to provide more detailed information about materials or techniques.

Address for Contacting the Author

Many journals give an address at the end of the paper (or in a footnote on the first page in some journals) where you can contact the author(s) for further information.

WHERE TO FIND RESEARCH EVENTS IN A RESEARCH REPORT

Chapter 3 described the sequence of events in research and indicated where they could be found in research reports. There is not a perfect correspondence between the research events and the sections of research reports, but it is easy to find the events in the report. The problem is introduced at the beginning and the specific purpose is stated by the end of the Introduction. The design is often summarized at the end of the Introduction or at the beginning of the Method section. Further details of the design are often incorporated in the description of the procedure. The procedures are described in the Method section. The method of data analysis is described separately in the Method section or at the beginning of the Results section, or is summarized as the results are reported in the Results section. Interpretations are presented in the Discussion section.

It may be helpful to go through an issue of the *Journal of Speech and Hearing Research* and find the research events in each research report. The easiest to locate should be the problem, purpose, procedure, and interpretation. The details of the design and the data analysis may be spread over more than one section.

EVALUATING RESEARCH REPORTS

If publication in a journal, monograph, or book ensured that the research reported was perfect in all respects, the authors' interpretation could be accepted at face value. The findings could be added to general knowledge, applied to practice, and used in designing further research. Perfection is rare in any type of research, though, and by its very nature, HCD research tends to be less perfect than basic research into normal human processes. Basic researchers test abstract theories of normal processes with easily available normal subjects and carefully controlled experimental techniques. HCD researchers confront the challenge of attempting to solve practical problems. They have to find representative subjects with HCDs, test or train them by whatever techniques are available, and control relevant variables as best they can. They cannot achieve perfection. It is important to evaluate their degree of success in order to decide how much their findings contribute to research, theory, and, practice.

As described in Chapter 2, there is a wide variety of HCDs. The aspects studied and the techniques used are continually changing. HCD researchers, like HCD practitioners, are necessarily self-taught in many respects. They do not usually work in a tidy, well-controlled laboratory.

Their research reports reflect the pioneering nature of their enterprise. Those who evaluate research reports for professional journals and books are themselves largely self-taught researchers who volunteer their time for the difficult task of reviewing the research of others. Under these circumstances, it is encouraging that published research reports are as good as they are.

Because HCD research is so difficult, diverse, and changeable, why should anyone other than researchers even attempt to evaluate research reports? It is the best way to learn about HCD research. By carefully evaluating each research event, readers can get a feeling for the challenge of HCD research. They can appreciate the usefulness of persisting in attempts to close important gaps in knowledge even though the theories, designs, procedures, and data analyses are not completely adequate for investigating the problem. If any published HCD study is carefully evaluated, shortcomings will be found. This is an inevitable result of attempting to answer practical questions.

General Strategies for Evaluating Research Reports

The evaluation of research reports requires an interesting type of research in itself. Readers must search through the sections of the report to discover the researcher's motives and plans, and chart their actions. Then they become the judges who evaluate the evidence. The first task is to find the research events. After evaluating each event, readers make an overall evaluation of the research report based on their knowledge of the topic. Research evaluation is a skill that is acquired only through practice. It requires background knowledge about research, theory, and practice. The critical attitude developed through evaluating research is essential for the professional who wants to meet the challenge of an ever-changing profession.

A potential stumbling block is lack of specialized knowledge about the problem and the usual methods of studying the problem. This can be avoided only by evaluating research reports within a particular field of interest. However, it is best not to completely restrict reading of research reports. Evaluating research reports on all aspects of HCDs is an excellent way for readers to broaden their knowledge about HCDs. This can be done by looking through all of the research reports in each issue of the *Journal of Speech and Hearing Research* and making a detailed evaluation of the research events in those papers that hold the most interest.

Readers should begin by seeing how much preliminary information can be obtained from the title and the abstract, and then work through the rest of the paper.

Evaluating the Problem, the Purpose, and the Design

The problem is always given in the first part of the Introduction, but it may not be divulged in full for a few paragraphs. The researchers should clearly relate the problem to a gap in knowledge about HCDs, but may not do so in studies concerning normal processes. There should be a description of accepted knowledge and theories concerning the problem, and a brief description of previous research directly related to the problem. If this information is not given, there is not an adequate basis for evaluating the contribution of the present study. Because of space limitations, readers may be referred to other publications for some of the essential information.

After the problem has been described, the purpose of the present research should be explicitly stated. This is done at the end of the Introduction in most research reports. When the purpose is stated, readers can evaluate the purpose to determine whether it seems sufficiently important and relevant to the problem. If the purpose is not specified, readers must review the rest of the report to infer what the purpose might have been. If the purpose cannot be determined, it will be difficult to judge the importance of the contribution to knowledge.

To evaluate the design, readers must discover where the essential details of the design have been described in the Introduction and Method sections. The design has to fit the purpose. Once the design is determined, the reader can evaluate it to determine whether it will obtain the information about the problem specified by the purpose. Specialized knowledge about research designs is required to evaluate the design.

Evaluating the Procedure

The exact operations for carrying out the design vary considerably from one research report to another. Care must be taken in evaluating each aspect of the procedure to make certain that independent and dependent variables have been adequately defined and relevant variables have been adequately controlled. This requires knowledge about theories, research methods, and practices relevant to the variables being investigated.

In evaluating subject selection, readers must determine how clearly the researchers defined the disorder, how representative the samples of subjects were of the total populations from which they were drawn, and whether groups of subjects were matched well enough on relevant variables. In evaluating assessment and training procedures, readers should decide whether the researchers have selected valid and reliable measures of the processes studied (see Chapters 4 and 8). In evaluating the remaining procedures, readers have to decide whether all relevant situation variables have been controlled, or whether the lack of control of relevant variables will confound the interpretation of the findings. In particular, readers must decide whether the subjects were adequately instructed and motivated, and whether the effects of practice, fatigue, and boredom were avoided.

Evaluating the Data Analysis

Evaluation of the data analysis depends on the method employed in the study. When traditional group methods have been used, it must be determined whether appropriate statistical techniques have been correctly applied. When other methods have been used, it must be determined whether methods appropriate to these analyses have been correctly applied.

Evaluating the Interpretation

The evaluation of the interpretation is crucial. It is first necessary to determine whether the researchers interpreted their findings in relation to the purpose of the study. Then the validity of the interpretation must be judged.

In research involving statistical analyses, a knowledge of statistics is necessary to determine whether the inferences concerning the statistical analyses are valid. It is not uncommon for researchers to conclude that the independent variables had significant effects when the statistical analyses do not permit such conclusions. It is even more common for the researchers to incorrectly conclude that a nonsignificant difference proves that there is no effect of an independent variable. The validity of the interpretation of studies that do not involve statistical analyses depends on the type of design and the accepted procedures for data analysis.

Most researchers are cautious in suggesting practical applications of the findings. When such suggestions are made, the evaluator has to decide whether this interpretation is really warranted. If the measures are not sufficiently direct, or the sample of subjects not sufficiently representative, or the results of the analyses not sufficiently definitive, suggested applications may be dangerously misleading. When there are suggestions for further research, readers might decide that other types of research might have even more value.

By the time the researchers present final conclusions at the end of the paper, readers should be prepared to reach final conclusions regarding the contribution of the research and to decide whether their conclusions agree with those of the researchers.

Final Suggestions Regarding Evaluation

Once the basic skills for evaluating the research have been developed, it is important to remember that all HCD researchers are doing the best they can with the tools at hand. Even when a study contains many imperfections, it may represent an effective strategy for obtaining as much of the desired information as possible. Not only must each research event be evaluated separately, but the total strategy of the researchers must be evaluated at the time of reaching a final conclusion concerning the contribution to knowledge.

Familiarity with the events of HCD research, as described in the preceding chapters, provides a necessary perspective for evaluating research. Skills for evaluating published research are built up by regularly reading published research with an informed critical attitude.

APPENDIX B

How to Plan, Carry Out, and Interpret HCD Research

All of the information given in the preceding chapters and in Appendix A is useful for planning, carrying out, and interpreting research. The more familiar researchers are with research methods that may be appropriate for the problem, the better the research will be.

THE REASONS FOR DOING RESEARCH

The reasons for doing the research are important. If the research is a student project, it cannot be too large a study in terms of design, procedure, data reduction, or data analysis. It may not be possible to meet all of the requirements for design and data analysis. Student projects should be restricted in scope, perhaps to simple group designs or case studies, and can be presented as exercises or preliminary studies.

For student theses, the research should be much more substantial. The research must meet the standards set for the thesis examination process, and should usually involve generally accepted approaches to a problem. When a student wishes to use an innovative approach, there should be careful consultation with the supervisor.

To learn how to do research, students doing projects or theses should make their own decisions concerning all aspects of the research whenever possible, and try to become experts on the topic. Students who rely on supervisors, statisticians, and others for decisions are not likely to become researchers who contribute important new information about HCDs.

For research that will be submitted for publication in research journals, the standards of the journals should be determined regarding numbers of subjects, types of designs, and data analyses. If there are too few subjects, flaws in the design, or inappropriate data analyses, there will be difficulty publishing the findings in a leading journal.

For research plans that will be submitted to government agencies, private foundations, or other sources to obtain funds needed for the research, it is very important to meet the standards set by the funding agency. The standards may vary considerably from one agency to another. Government agencies usually set very precise criteria for the importance of the problem, the thoroughness of the review of relevant literature, the number and type of subjects, the appropriateness of the design and data analysis, and the approval of an ethics committee. Private foundations may use less strict criteria, but may support a more restricted type of research. Researchers should familiarize themselves with the exact research criteria and with the exact type of research funded before writing proposals for funding. A great deal of time and effort may be expended for nothing if researchers do not pay sufficient attention to these important details.

If the research is based on previous research by the present researchers or others, all of the details of the previous research should be reviewed in designing the present research. This should be done in as critical a manner as possible. There may be relevant research, theories, or practical issues that were not considered in previous research, perhaps because they involve new information. Improvements in the designs or analyses may be possible, or alternative approaches may provide fresh perspectives. If there is sufficient information about a problem from past research, the researchers have to plan research that will provide an important confirmation or a significant extension of the previous findings.

If preliminary or exploratory research is undertaken, researchers should use their imagination, ingenuity, and previous knowledge to the fullest. The first study on a problem should be broad enough in scope to suggest the most promising directions for further research.

TYPE OF RESEARCH

Another important planning consideration is the type of research, which will depend on both the interests and inclinations of the researchers. Researchers usually restrict their interests to one field (for example, audiology, education of children who are hearing impaired, or speech–language pathology), to one type of disorder within the field (for example, peripheral auditory disorders or speech disorders), and in some cases to one aspect of one disorder (for example, tongue movements in stutterers). To the extent that there is accepted knowledge as opposed to guesswork concerning the disorders studied, research planning can be solidly based on previous knowledge. Research on broader aspects of communication will tend to involve less definite knowledge. Some researchers may prefer to work on more definite problems, and others on problems where the frontiers of knowledge are uncharted.

RESEARCH APPROACH

Once the type of research is selected, researchers have to decide on the approach. In most cases, approaches used by previous researchers for similar problems will be selected. Quantitative approaches using standard designs and statistical analyses are selected for most HCD problems. However, for problems involving broader aspects of communication, qualitative approaches using innovative methods may be selected. There is a tendency for most researchers studying peripheral processes to use quantitative, analytic approaches, and for some researchers studying more central processes to use qualitative approaches.

Researchers must decide whether to use group designs or individual subject designs. Group designs are still most common in the *Journal of Speech and Hearing Research,* but other designs are often useful. Case studies may be used in the early stages of research on a problem. Single subject designs may be used if the researchers have definite hypotheses about an effective form of intervention. Observational methods may be most appropriate for studying communicative interactions of small numbers of subjects.

The choice of approach depends not only on the type of problem, but also on the potential advantages and disadvantages of each approach. Quantitative approaches tend to yield definite but limited knowledge. Qualitative approaches tend to yield unlimited but indefinite information. Studies of individuals provide detailed and definite information, but are difficult to generalize. Researchers who are seriously concerned with the choice of approach can find arguments for and against each type of approach. However, HCD researchers tend to be more concerned with the achievement of useful knowledge than with the exact approach used.

COLLABORATIVE RESEARCH

Research may be carried out by pairs of students, a student and supervisor, a student and thesis committee, pairs of researchers, teams of researchers, or one solitary researcher. Chance plays a part in the effectiveness of each form of collaboration. Different persons have different talents. Some are best at suggesting ideas for research, and others at searching the literature, making effective designs, planning and carrying out procedures, analyzing data, or interpreting the results. Collaboration can be useful for arriving at common decisions at each stage of research, or for allowing collaborators to be responsible for the parts that suit their talents. Those who want to be able to function as independent, self-sufficient researchers should participate in all aspects of research.

GENERAL STRATEGY

Thoughtfulness is the watchword for each stage of planning, carrying out, and interpreting research. Research requires a large intellectual and emotional investment. Every effort should be made to avoid hasty decisions, easy solutions, and convenient shortcuts. Poorly conceived, executed, and interpreted research is embarrassing for everyone concerned, and will not increase knowledge about HCDs.

Researchers have to proceed in a thoughtful, responsible manner with the realization that they cannot know everything about the problem, research designs, procedures, and methods of data analysis. They must learn as much as they can and then do the best they can. Those who find HCD research a formidable prospect should begin by choosing straightforward problems that can be studied by orderly methods.

The potential rewards for researchers are great. Some of the most important advances in science have been made by clever students who bring a fresh perspective to a problem. Appropriate training and hard work are necessary elements. Chance plays an unavoidable role, or else research would not be research. The final ingredient is thoughtfulness.

HOW TO START

If researchers do not have a pressing problem that demands investigation, there are several ways of finding one. Obvious approaches are to read relevant literature concerning research, theory, and practice; and to consult researchers, theorists, and practitioners. Another strategy is to keep a list of problems as they come to mind, and then get the opinions of others concerning their potential importance. Some problems that seem very important at first do not stand up to later scrutiny.

Once a potential problem or problems have emerged, possible approaches can be considered. Is it a large problem that requires extensive planning, a smaller study that can be carried out with limited resources, or a new idea that requires preliminary exploration? This is a stage at which time must be set aside for thoughtful reflection as opposed to impulsive decision making, or the researchers may find themselves launched on an unsuccessful enterprise. Advice may be sought at this stage from those who use different approaches.

At some point, a decision is made to proceed further with the problem. Then the research is under way, at least in a preliminary manner, and the next stages of planning can proceed.

REVIEW OF THE LITERATURE

After a possible problem has been selected, the exact purpose of research on the problem cannot be determined without a thorough search of the literature. The best strategy is to find the most recent publications concerning the problem, particularly reviews of research and theory. This can be done by reading current issues of the *Journal of Speech and Hearing Research* and other appropriate journals, looking through reference sources such as *Current Contents*, writing to researchers who have studied the problem, and using computer search procedures such as *Medline* and *PsycInfo*. As information is gathered, the current status of both theories and research should be carefully evaluated to define an important gap in knowledge concerning the problem.

PLANNING THE RESEARCH

When the literature has been reviewed, the purpose can be defined in relation to an important gap in knowledge. Then further planning of the design, procedure, and analysis can proceed. If the original purpose cannot be carried out because of limitations imposed by the design, procedure, or analysis, it is modified accordingly.

Once a tentative purpose has been defined, there is a temptation to select an obvious design. It is best to take the time to consider a variety of designs before reaching a final decision. This is where a team of researchers and consultants with different experience and viewpoints regarding research designs can be helpful. An essential aspect of this phase of planning is the identification of independent variables, dependent variables, and relevant variables that must be controlled.

When a design has been tentatively selected, the researchers must determine whether an acceptable procedure can be formulated. The first considerations are whether subjects are available in sufficient numbers, and whether relevant variables can be defined and controlled. If the variables to be studied are not well defined, it may be difficult to decide on valid and reliable procedures for assessing or manipulating the variables. Needs for equipment, facilities, and technical assistance must be carefully considered to determine whether available resources are sufficient. If not, assistance must be sought from outside sources.

If qualitative methods are used, data analyses may be planned as the data are being collected. If quantitative group designs are used, methods of data analysis should be selected before final decisions are reached concerning the purpose, design, and procedure. Such forethought seems to go against human nature. Even experienced researchers may not explicitly plan the data analysis until the data have been collected. However, there are two important dangers in not planning the data analysis ahead of time. First, the choice of analyses may be biased by an examination of the data. Such bias makes the probability estimates obtained by statistical analysis meaningless and invalidates the contribution to knowledge about HCDs. Second, if the data analysis methods are not selected in advance, the researchers may find that their data do not meet the requirements of the available methods of analysis. In such a case, the data will be uninterpretable and will not contribute to knowledge about HCDs. In addition to avoiding the above dangers, planning the data analysis at the time of designing the study can have an important advantage. Researchers may be able to make planned comparisons on the basis of previous knowledge and theories, and thus increase the chances of a contribution to knowledge about HCDs.

Once the best possible adjustments of the plan have been made to integrate the purpose, design, procedure, and analysis, a final plan can be decided on. At this point the researchers should take the time to review the plan to determine whether there have been any oversights, or whether any alternative approaches have suggested themselves. The final outcome of the research should be carefully considered. In adjusting their plans for the separate parts, researchers may lose sight of how their findings are intended to contribute useful knowledge about HCDs.

PRELIMINARY STUDIES

If there has been little or no previous research on a problem, the researchers may not be able to tell in advance whether their plan will result in usable data. For example, if an experimental task has not been used before with subjects with HCDs, the researchers may not be certain that the subjects will understand the task. The task may be too difficult for HCD subjects, resulting in floor effects, or too easy for control subjects, resulting in ceiling effects. In such cases, a small preliminary study can be very helpful in planning the exact procedures that will be used. Pilot studies are also helpful when researchers are applying for funds for research on a new topic for which previous research cannot be cited. Granting agencies are never as optimistic as the researchers themselves about the chances of a contribution to knowledge.

DATA COLLECTION

When the final plan is put into action, the data are collected. Data collection must take place exactly as planned. Otherwise, the data may be meaningless or misleading. The data have to be collected in a careful manner. The researchers must assure themselves that those who gather the data are reliable and conscientious, especially when the data are gathered in an unsupervised situation. The researchers themselves must have a responsible attitude toward their research. Anyone who collects data in a careless manner may harm themselves, their profession, and persons with HCDs.

DATA ANALYSIS

When data analyses have been preplanned, they must be carried out according to plan. Great care should be taken to calculate and display descriptive statistics that reveal the salient features of the data. Such displays can take the forms of graphs or tables. Great care should also be taken in presenting the results of complex analyses such as higher order interactions, multivariate correlation analyses, meta-analyses, and path analyses.

When data are qualitatively analyzed, the analysis may take place as part of the data collection, and should proceed according to the established conventions of the qualitative method.

INTERPRETATION

The researchers' job is not finished when the data have been collected. It is their responsibility to determine the extent to which the purpose has been achieved, to relate the findings to previous research, and to describe the contribution to knowledge. Whereas the previous research events have required a great deal of deductive reasoning, the interpretation requires inductive reasoning. The researchers have to determine the implications of the findings as well as understand the findings themselves. Then the interpretation can be extended to suitably cautious recommendations regarding practical applications, and useful suggestions can be made regarding the most promising directions for further research.

When the researchers have found an important problem and given their most thoughtful attention to each phase of planning, data collection, and data analysis, the interpretation is the culmination of their work.

FUNDING

When an extensive research program is planned, or when a particular project involves large expenses, the researchers may have to obtain a relatively large amount of money in order to complete the research. This requires the preparation and submission of a research grant application. A great deal of time and effort is required to prepare applications. They have to be done in a certain form, and a great deal of information must be presented in a limited amount of space.

A potential drawback for those considering applying for research funding is that the chances of being funded may be small, especially if a nontraditional approach or a controversial topic is involved. Many researchers may hesitate to devote their time to a doubtful enterprise. Some researchers may lack the patience to follow the rigid formats of applications, and some may resent the idea that their choice of research is dictated by its potential acceptability to a funding agency.

These are important considerations, but there are also potential benefits of applying for funds. The researchers are forced to do thoughtful planning at each stage—to select an important problem, present a succinct literature review, define an explicit purpose, choose an appropriate design, attend to all details of procedure, and preplan the data analysis. Having done this, they have the advantage of the peer review process. The application is reviewed by experts in their field, and even if it is not funded, the researchers are provided with the critical comments of the reviewers. This free advice can be worth a great deal to the researchers in suggesting how the research plan could be improved. Then the researchers may be successful in further efforts to obtain funds.

ETHICAL CONSIDERATIONS

Ethical considerations in HCD research relate to the researchers' responsibility to plan, carry out, and report the findings of research in a responsible manner, and to deal with subjects in an ethical manner. The institutions that employ researchers and the agencies that grant them funds require that all research proposals be reviewed by an ethics committee to guarantee that ethical procedures will be used. These include not exposing subjects to physical or psychological risks, obtaining informed consent from subjects (and, where necessary, parents and teachers), not deceiving subjects regarding the purpose of the research, and not divulging private information about the subjects. Standard forms are required for obtaining the informed consent of subjects and for certifying the approval of an ethics committee. Researchers have to be aware of ethical considerations in planning research and take the necessary steps to insure that ethical requirements have been met. Unethical practices with regard to the treatment of subjects and to the research itself can have grave consequences for all concerned. Similar ethical considerations apply to animal research. A few unethical researchers can cast suspicion on the whole research enterprise and prevent the carrying out of research that might be of great benefit to persons with human communication disorders. Information about ethical considerations in HCD research is given in a section called Research Subjects in "Information for Authors" at the end of each issue of the *Journal of Speech and Hearing Research*.

COMPLETING RESEARCH

After reading the preceding chapters, the preceding appendix, and this appendix, it should be obvious that a great deal of thought, study, and effort must go into any research, no matter how modest. Many different skills must be brought to bear before the research can be completed. The final product cannot be a perfunctory effort—it must be a useful contribution to knowledge. Unfortunately, many research projects are never brought to the final stage of completion. Like many other worthwhile enterprises, research requires sustained effort, a drive for completion, and a useful product. Anyone who does not feel equal to the challenge should think very seriously before undertaking research. For those who accept the challenge, the rewards can provide lifelong satisfaction, and can be of benefit to many future generations of persons with HCDs.

Research is not completed until it is available in published form. Appendix C describes this final phase of research.

APPENDIX C

How to Write Research Reports

The final outcome of most research is a research report. This may take a number of different forms, such as oral presentations at seminars and professional meetings, theses, monographs, chapters, and books. The traditional form of contribution to knowledge is submission of a research report for publication in a professional journal. The report is reviewed by journal editors and expert consultants. If they recommend acceptance, the report is published and becomes a formal contribution to knowledge. They may also recommend revision and resubmission, or rejection. The care taken in planning, carrying out, and interpreting the research, as described in Appendix B, will largely determine the chances for acceptance and publication.

Suggestions for writing a research report for publication in a professional journal are given first because the requirements for published reports are the most standard and rigorous. Then suggestions are given for other forms of report, including student projects, theses, and reports intended for oral presentation.

GENERAL WRITING STYLE

Several basic rules should be followed regarding the writing style for research reports:

1. Practice makes perfect. Writing style should improve with each research report, providing writers make a conscious effort to improve.

2. Researchers should revise everything they write. Most professional writers make endless revisions. Amateurs cannot expect to get it right the first, second, or even the third time.

3. Researchers should ask others (fellow students, supervisors, colleagues) to make comments and suggestions after they have completed a draft of the report. The most valuable suggestions may come from persons who have published a number of research reports themselves. They should be asked to be as critical as if they were reviewing the report for publication in a professional journal. This can be a great help in achieving an effective writing style.

4. Researchers should find a person who has written clear and concise research reports on the same general topic, and use this person's writing as a model until they have developed an effective style of their own.

SPECIFIC WRITING STYLE

Each journal has its own style, and style requirements are usually given at the beginning or the end of each journal issue. For the *Journal of Speech and Hearing Research*, there is a page at the end of each issue headed "Information for Authors." Instructions are given regarding the type of research reports published in the journal, the procedure for reviewing reports submitted, the number of copies to be submitted, the manuscript style, and ethical considerations. The *Journal of Speech and Hearing Research*, like many other journals, requires that papers follow the style specified in the APA manual (*Publication Manual of the American Psychological Association*). This manual gives specific instructions for preparing each part of the report, plus general suggestions about writing style, grammar, and other useful information. It is the best style manual of its type and is highly recommended for anyone who prepares research reports. The APA manual can be purchased from the Order Department, APA, PO Box 2710, Hyattsville, MD 20784.

Of particular relevance to HCD research are the APA guidelines to reduce bias in language. Authors are advised to avoid constructions that might imply bias against persons on the basis of gender, sexual orientation, racial or ethnic group, age, or disability. In talking about people with disabilities, the person should always be mentioned first, to avoid equating the person with the disability. For example, "children with language disorders" is preferable to "language disordered children."

If there is any doubt concerning style, researchers should consult the journal to which the report is to be submitted. They should look through a current issue to find an example of the aspect of style in question. While writing the paper, it is best to find a similar report for use as a model in the journal to which the report will be submitted. The report should be of good quality in both content and style.

CONTENT

Information concerning the content of research reports can be obtained by consulting the APA manual and a current issue of the journal to which the report is to be submitted.

Title

The title briefly describes the research, almost always in 15 words or less.

Authors

Authors are usually listed in the order of the importance of their contribution to the research. Research assistants and technicians who carried out instructions but did not contribute to decision making are usually not included as coauthors.

Abstract

The report begins with an abstract of the study in 150 words or less. The abstract usually describes the problem, purpose, and design in about one sentence each, and the procedure, results, and discussion in one or two sentences each.

Introduction

The introduction is the first section of the written report, and usually has no heading. It may range from about 250 words (one double-spaced typewritten page) to 1,500 words (six double-spaced typewritten pages). As described in the preceding chapters and appendixes, the introduction should succinctly describe research, theory, and practice relevant to the problem, the problem itself, and the specific purpose. The design is often summarized at the end of the introduction.

Method

The method section is usually relatively long because it contains subsections describing the subjects, equipment, materials, and procedures. An introductory paragraph describing the design and a final subsection describing the data analysis may also be included. Enough details must be given for other researchers to repeat the study.

Results

The results present the data gathered in the study, plus the results of data analyses. The writing of the results section is part of the research itself, because decisions regarding the final organization and presentation of the findings are often not made until the results section is written. Authors should make every effort to present all the data that may be useful to readers. A great deal of care should be taken in deciding what data to include and in preparing tables and figures. When sufficient information is given in the proper form, readers who are familiar with the research topic can often interpret the findings for themselves. As researchers become experienced in critically evaluating published research and in searching the literature for topics of interest, they will see the value of a clear and detailed presentation of results.

Discussion

The interpretation of results in the discussion section tends to be quite variable in length, style, and content. There may be a combined results and discussion section, a separate discussion section with or without subsections, or several final sections with specific headings such as Considerations for Future Studies and Conclusions. Even more than with the results section, the writing of the discussion section is usually part of the research itself. The writers often do not arrive at a final interpretation of their findings until they have to write the discussion section.

The style of the discussion section may vary from a very narrow operational description of the results to a lengthy, far-reaching interpretation. Usually the main findings are summarized and related to the purpose at the beginning of the section. Then, limitations imposed by the design, procedure, and analysis are considered, and the findings are related to previous research and theory. Finally, recommendations may be made for practical applications and further research, and general conclusions may be stated.

The writing of the discussion should involve the most thought, the greatest care, and the most revisions. It sums up the writers' contribution to knowledge. As can be seen by reading research reports, sometimes the contribution is a small, specific increment of knowledge that can be briefly and succinctly described; sometimes the writers extensively interpret complex findings; and sometimes they use all of their eloquence to persuade readers of the importance of a new approach or a new topic. This section is usually the most difficult to write, but it is the authors' opportunity to put the final touches to a lasting contribution to knowledge. The manner in which results are interpreted is an important factor in determining the impact of the report and the frequency with which the research is cited in subsequent reports.

Acknowledgments

In a brief section following the discussion, the writers should acknowledge help received from colleagues in planning and writing, from representatives of institutions in making subjects and facilities available, and from granting agencies for providing funds for the research.

References

References must be cited in the text of the article in a standard manner, and a list of references must be given after the acknowledgments, also in a standard manner. The exact reference style may vary from one journal to another. All references in the text and the reference list should be double- and triple-checked for exact accuracy. Incorrect references are very obvious to the experts whom the writers of the paper most wish to impress.

Appendixes

Details of tests and other technical information that might be of use to readers can be presented in appendixes after the references.

OVERALL WRITING STRATEGIES

It is not necessary to write the sections of the research report in the order in which they will appear. If there are several authors, they may share the task and write the sections that suit their abilities and interests. If there is a single author, the sections can be written as it suits the author's convenience. For beginning writers, the first step may be to assemble a folder of notes concerning each section. Whenever there is a pertinent thought or a specific detail that could be reported, it can be put on a piece of paper and stored in the folder. At some point, a draft of the section can be written on the basis of the notes. The draft should be revised several times until an acceptable first draft has been completed. In this manner a complete draft can be assembled for comments and suggestions by research collaborators, fellow students, supervisors, or colleagues.

A convenient order of writing sections for beginning researchers may be to make a rough, perhaps overlong draft of the introduction, and a more careful draft of the method section. Then a thoughtful draft of the results should be written. While this is being done, the writer should assemble notes for the discussion. At the time of beginning the discussion there may be a lack of interpretive ideas to add to the bare facts of the results. Prior notes can be very useful. It is also helpful to think about the interpretation whenever there is an opportunity for reflection. Often the final stage of writing is completion of the introduction.

Regardless of the strategies used for writing drafts, the paper should be revised on the basis of whatever critical suggestions can be obtained until it is in a clear, brief, orderly form suitable for publication. Once again, the best model for the proper final form is a good paper on a similar topic.

REVISION AFTER REVIEW BY JOURNAL

After the researchers have prepared the best report they can and submitted it to a journal, they must wait for several months to get the reaction of the reviewers. In rare instances, the editor will accept the paper exactly as submitted, with no revisions required. More often, a paper will be accepted with the condition that certain specific parts be revised on the basis of the reviewers' suggestions. In some cases the authors may be asked to resubmit a greatly revised or completely rewritten paper for a second review. Finally, the editor may inform the writers that the paper is not suitable for publication in the journal. The editor usually sends the comments of the reviewers to the authors.

Beginning writers should not be overwhelmed by critical comments of reviewers. Although the comments may seem at first to be cruel, unfair, and devastating, they can be of great value. They are free advice given by experts on the topic of the research. If the paper is accepted with minor revisions, the writers should cheerfully make revisions that do not change the meaning of the paper. For any suggestions that they disagree with, they should send a detailed statement of their reasons for rejecting the suggestion along with the revised manuscript.

Less fortunate authors who are required to make major revisions and resubmit the paper for a second review should do so whenever they feel that the criticisms are justified and that they are capable of making the required revisions. If they decide not to revise and resubmit, they may wish to submit the paper to another journal with different or less rigorous standards. For HCD research, however, the papers that receive the greatest attention and respect are those published in the *Journal of Speech and Hearing Research* and other leading journals. Authors should try to swallow their pride, overcome their distaste for making yet one more revision, and do their best to put their paper into an acceptable form.

If a paper is rejected, authors may wish to submit it elsewhere, or they may accept the editor's verdict that it is not worthy of publication. It is not wise to react by abandoning the research entirely. Reviewers usually have a good perspective, and their criticisms can be used to plan research that will be accepted for publication. If researchers are using a new research approach or a new technique for assessment or training, the reviewers' rejections may seem biased against innovations that overthrow traditional methods. Some reviewers tenaciously guard "accepted" theories, methods, and techniques in what seems to be a narrow and dogmatic manner, and thus impede new approaches that may contribute important information. In such cases researchers are perhaps best advised to find a journal more sympathetic to the new approach. Publication of obviously important research in other journals can lead to acceptance by the "mainstream" professional journals.

READING THE PROOF

When a paper has been accepted for publication, the authors will eventually receive a "proof" of the paper as it will appear in the journal, and be asked to carefully read it, note any errors, and immediately return it. The authors may be tempted to scan the paper rapidly and return it, having read it carefully too many times already. However, a careful proofreading in the manner recommended by the APA manual is an absolute necessity. Both small errors such as misspelled words and major errors such as omitted paragraphs or incorrectly labeled figures are easy to miss with cursory proofreading. They will come back to haunt the authors. Nothing is worse than to see an otherwise excellent paper riddled with errors, especially when they distort the findings.

PREPARING OTHER TYPES OF RESEARCH REPORT

Other types of research report may require somewhat different writing styles.

Student Research Projects

Student research projects are usually acceptable when written in the style of the *Journal of Speech and Hearing Research*, following the guidelines of the APA manual, unless a specific style is required by the research supervisor. The main differences concern the length of sections. The introduction may be longer, with a more detailed review of previous research. More detailed descriptions of methods and results may be given, with lengthy appendices where necessary. The discussion should be long enough to demonstrate the student's understanding of the results and ability to interpret them in a creative manner. Otherwise the student project report can closely follow the standard format. Reports of student research projects are usually considerably shorter than student theses.

Student Theses

Students should consult the regulations of their university, as well as their thesis supervisor, regarding the recommended style for master's and doctoral theses. A thesis is usually much longer than published research reports and student research projects. The sections may be divided into several chapters. Following the introduction, there is a lengthy review of the literature, sometimes divided into more than one section or chapter. Methods are described in detail, as are results. The discussion chapter must demonstrate the student's ability to understand and interpret research, and should clearly indicate the contribution to knowledge of the thesis research. A thesis on a similar topic that received a very good rating from the student's department can be used as a model.

Some universities permit students to modify the standard format by submitting research that has already been published as papers, monographs, book chapters, or books, along with a detailed review of the literature and a detailed interpretation.

Monographs

Monographs are reports of research that cannot be adequately presented within the page limits of a journal article. They often describe a series of studies rather than a single study. Thesis research may involve too much information for a single journal article, and be published as a series of articles or a monograph. Monographs usually follow standard journal style. Authors take special care in the preparation of monographs, because they can be very substantial contributions to knowledge.

Book Chapters

Research may be reported in the form of book chapters that report findings that have been presented at a conference or symposium. Or, the book editor may wish to assemble a number of research reports on a particular topic. The chapter may report more than one study and may report research plans and preliminary results of incomplete research. Research reports in book chapters may be less rigorous than research reports in journals. Authors are more free to speculate about preliminary findings. However, careless speculation not supported by later research is not a useful contribution to knowledge. If there is no careful review of submissions, authors of book chapters must be responsible themselves for the quality of their research report.

Books

Books are very ambitious undertakings, often requiring several years for completion. Authors usually submit a preliminary outline to several publishers and sign a contract for the book before completing the final writing. Some research projects or series of studies, including student theses, merit publication in book form. Authors are more free to report the research in whatever style they wish. Publishers usually ask experts to review the final manuscript more for content than for style. Then copy editors help the author put the book in final form.

Oral Presentations

Unpublished research is often reported in oral presentations at departmental seminars and professional conferences. The style of such presentations depends on the time limitations. If the time is limited to 10 or 15 minutes, the author should write the talk in advance and carefully rehearse it until it can be presented with proper timing and intonation. If it is one of a series of presentations, only highlights that can be easily understood should be presented.

The problem should be briefly stated, with a very brief review of previous research. The main details of the method should be presented slowly and carefully, with appropriate audiovisual aids. Only the main details of the results that can be immediately understood by the audience should be presented. Great care should be taken with audiovisual aids to present the salient features of the findings in clear visual and audible form. Comments on audiovisual displays should be carefully rehearsed. Unrehearsed descriptions of the data in tables and figures always result in the speaker exceeding the time limit, to the great discomfort of the audience. The final conclusions should be brief and to the point.

Carefully prepared and rehearsed presentations are a credit to the speakers and to the institution they represent, and are well worth the time and effort expended in preparation. These recommendations apply equally to presentations at oral defenses of theses, which are usually about 15 to 20 minutes long.

Presentations longer than 20 minutes may be written out in advance, or presented more informally, depending on the speaker's preference. Beginning researchers may need to make formal presentations. However, there is a danger of losing the attention of the audience if the talk is read in an uninflected voice and gives details of interest only to the speaker. Once again, the more practice, the better. The speaker should consciously attempt to develop effective strategies for lengthy research presentations. Less gifted speakers may take years to develop an effective style.

WORD PROCESSORS

Word processors are invaluable for the preparation of research reports. The separate sections of the reports can be kept in separate files. References can be added and deleted as needed. If graphic presentations are important, special software is available. Revisions of drafts and revisions of the final manuscript in response to reviewers' comments are easily done. Every aspect of writing is immeasurably facilitated.

APPENDIX D

Answers to Exercises

CHAPTER 4

1. a. Subject controls: age, gender, linguistic background, vocabulary knowledge

   Situation controls: listening conditions, instructions, task

   b. Failure to control age, gender, linguistic background, or vocabulary knowledge

   c. Independent: speech production (phonological) disorders

   Dependent: performance on speech perception test

   d. Phonological disorder, no phonological disorder

   e. Internal validity: relevant subject and situation variables controlled

   External validity: performance on speech perception test reflects speech perception abilities in real-life situation

   f. Repeat test, compare scores on halves of test, compare scores on alternate forms of test

   g. No: with a pointing response, observer reliability is not a problem

2. a. Independent variable: training

   Dependent variable: fluency on speech samples

  b. Before training and after training

  c. Relation of fluency on speech sample to fluency in natural communicative situations

  d. Assess observer reliability by determining percentage of agreement of two observers in judging fluency on speech samples

3. a. Independent variable: training

   Dependent variable: fluency on speech samples

  b. Training, no training

  c. Subject controls: age, gender, education, severity of stuttering, history of treatment

   Situation controls: instructions, method of recording speech sample, training procedure

  d. The untrained group

  e. Failure to match groups in severity of stuttering

CHAPTER 5

1. One independent variable, two levels of independent variable, one dependent variable

2. The desirable minimum is 20 (10 per group) and the absolute minimum is 10 (5 per group)

3. (1) natural group, (2) repeated measurement, (3) matched group

4. Personality problems: combined matched and natural group

   Speech aid: repeated measurement or matched group

   Speech discrimination tests: repeated measurement

5. Independent variable: hearing aids

   Levels of the independent variable: standard and new hearing aids

Dependent variable: a measure of hearing (e.g., pure tone test)

Subject controls: age, gender, amount and type of hearing loss

Situation controls: listening situation, hearing test

Random assignment design: randomly assign subjects to two groups from available population of hearing impaired. Test one aid with each group

Matched group design: match two groups from available population of individuals with hearing impairment in terms of age, gender, amount and type of hearing loss; test one aid with each group

Repeated measurement design: select a representative group of individuals with hearing impairment from available population. Test both aids with the entire group; counterbalance order of presentation of aids by testing half of the subjects with one aid first and the other half with the other aid first

CHAPTER 6

1. a. 2 × 2 repeated measures factorial design

   Independent variables: background noise (quiet and noise), word context (isolated words, words in sentences)

   Dependent variable: performance on word recognition test

   Minimum subjects: 20 to 40

   Order of presentation of background noise and of word context must be counterbalanced

   Example of interaction: the effects of noise as compared with quiet are greater for words in isolation than for words in sentences

   b. Independent group design with more than two levels

   Independent variable: age (age 1, age 2, age 3, etc.)

   Dependent variable: performance on speech perception test

Minimum number of subjects: 5 to 10 per level

No counterbalancing or interaction

c. 2 × 2 independent group design

Independent variables: voice disorder (voice disorder, no voice disorder), gender

Dependent variable: judgment of speech intelligibility from speech sample

Minimum number of subjects: 20 to 40

No counterbalancing required

Example of interaction: the difference between normal female subjects and those with voice disorders is smaller than the difference between two such groups of male subjects

d. Repeated measurement design with more than two levels

Independent variable: background noise (quiet, low noise, moderate noise, etc.)

Dependent variable: performance on speech perception test

Minimum number of subjects: 5 to 10 per level

Counterbalance order of background noise

No interaction

e. 2 × 2 mixed factorial design

Independent variables: voice disorder (voice disorder, no voice disorder), phoneme class (vowels, consonants)

Dependent variable: judged intelligibility of vowels and consonants in a standardized speech sample

Minimum number of subjects: 20 to 40

No counterbalancing necessary (vowels and consonants evenly distributed in speech sample)

Example of interaction: difference between voice disorder and no voice disorder groups is greatest for vowels

CHAPTER 12

1. a. Main effects: Hearing aids (Aid 1, Aid 2),

     Noise (quiet, noise)

   Interaction: Hearing Aids × Noise

   b. Main effects: Age (young, older)

     Gender (girls, boys)

     Task (picture description, story retelling)

   Interactions: Age × Gender

     Age × Task

     Gender × Task

     Age × Gender × Task

   c. Main effects: Age (young, older)

     Education (high school, university)

     Amount of training (0 weeks, 4 weeks, 8 weeks)

     Amount of hearing loss (moderate, severe)

   Interactions: Age × Education

     Age × Training

     Age × Hearing

     Education × Training

     Education × Hearing

     Training × Hearing

     Age × Education × Training

     Age × Education × Hearing

     Education × Training × Hearing

     Age × Education × Training × Hearing

2. a. There is better speech discrimination with Hearing Aid 1 in quiet, and with Hearing 2 in noise.

   b. Younger boys, older boys, and older girls make more errors in story retelling than in picture description. Older girls make the same amount of errors in story retelling and picture description.

   c. All groups show continued improvement with training from 4 weeks to 8 weeks except the younger, university educated group with moderate hearing loss, who reach maximum performance in 4 weeks.

   (Note: The easiest examples of higher order interactions are those in which one cell shows a different trend for a main effect, as illustrated by the example of a 2 × 2 × 2 interaction in the text.)

INDEX

About the Author

Donald Doehring is Professor Emeritus, School of Communication Sciences and Disorders, McGill University, Montreal, Canada. He has done a great deal of research and published extensively on hearing, language, and reading disorders in children and adults. For more than 25 years he taught a course on research methods in human communication disorders.